Flying Wi__
Broken Wing

By Sat Mehta

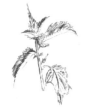

Nettle Books

Published 2012 by Nettle Books
nettlebooks@hotmail.co.uk

ISBN: 978-0-9561513-2-2

Classification: Biography

Foreword

by Dickie Bird

World Cricket Test Umpire

I first met Sat Mehta in April 1987. I had just returned from umpiring World Test Match cricket in Delhi, Mumbai, Chennai and Kolkata.

I sought his professional opinion about a condition that troubles many a visitor to India, on account of the dust and dry air. As I had spent six weeks touring the sub-continent from top to bottom, I reckoned that if anyone should know the answer to combating the effects of a foreign climate, he would.

Sat and I have remained friends ever since. His love of cricket must go back nearly as far as mine! I sent out a special invitation to Sat and his wife to come to my final test match, England v India at Lord's. They came to see me in the Hilton Hotel afterwards. He has been to many cricket matches umpired by me and was also present at the unveiling of my statue, which stands virtually on the spot where I was born in Barnsley in 1933.

It is with enormous pleasure that I write the foreword to this book. I hope you enjoy reading Sat's personal account of growing up in a land that has given the world so many great cricketers.

Dickie Bird, February 2012

Dedicated to my children,
Louise, Paul, Clare & Jane,
and to my grandchildren,
Sara, Molly and Holly.
They are the future

Contents

1: Exodus

THE BRITISH QUIT INDIA in 1947, leaving the sub-continent in a state of total chaos. At that time I was five years old and lived with my family in the town of Kamalia, in the Punjab region. This part of India saw the worst of the bloodshed.

Ali Jinnah, the leader of the Muslim League, did not share Mahatma Gandhi's vision of an undivided India and wanted the top of India to form a country where only Muslims would live. The new country was to be near our family farmlands. The border was finally decided upon and it cut between the Punjab's two major cities, Lahore and Amritsar. Tension between Hindus and Muslims simmered and outbreaks of violence were frequent. The British dissolved their administration and left on 15th August. The violence escalated and suddenly full-blown civil war erupted everywhere in our region.

"Kill 'im, kill 'im!!" the crowd roared. Uncle Bodhraj Mehta was dragged into the market place and repeatedly stabbed in the chest until he died. Surinder, his wife, was held back from going to his aid by my *Bauji* (my Father) and Grandfather. She looked on helplessly as Bodhraj lay in the dust, a pool of bright red blood pumping from his chest, soaking his shirt and spreading like a river, onto the ground around him.

"Mehtas, we're coming for all of you!" The mob then went on the rampage and set about torching everything Hindus owned. The raid began from the town hall. Muslims rounded up Hindus and Sikhs in the marketplace and killed them. Surinder knew some of the mob. They had worked for her and Bodhraj on the farm. "How can they do this to us?" she screamed. She wanted to confront them. She wanted to shoot them. Indoors, Sunil, their four-year-old son, was unaware his father lay dead in the marketplace.

Bauji hurried under cover of darkness to his father's house and hammered on the door. Grandfather pulled him in, saying "Come in for God's sake. I've got Surinder and Sunil here. I couldn't let them stay alone." Like the rest of us, uncle Bodhraj's family had been living peacefully in a Muslim area. Bodhraj had been a leader of the local council in Kamalia and was an administrator and tax collector for the British government.

Grandfather and Bauji went to the town square to bring back Bodhraj's body, which lay where it had fallen. Bauji yelled to anyone listening: "For pity's sake, let's at least have his body for cremation. What good's he to you now?" That evening the body of my uncle was cremated without fuss at the back of the house. The funeral pyre was lit by his father and his brother. Grandfather Mehta's house and compound were big and the buildings were made of strong brick, so Bauji gathered friends and relations in Grandfather's house. They organised a patrol day and night. Armed with revolvers, double-barreled shotguns used for hunting, and large *lathi* bamboo sticks, they managed to hold the compound for a few nights.

That night the mob gathered around the house. We saw the flicker of the torches and heard them scream: *"Mehtas! Come out, bastards! You're all bloody cowards!"* and *"Get out! The place doesn't belong to you!"* This carried on for an hour, and then suddenly the mob melted away into the shadows as an army truck rolled up. After that night, we all wanted to leave.

Mobs patrolled the streets, shouting: *"Kill Sikh, kill Hindu, kill, kill, kill!"* and *"Pakistan jindabab! Long live Pakistan!"* To save their lives, many Sikhs and Hindus converted to Islam. We heard that terrible atrocities had been committed by marauding gangs. Rumours flew back and forth that Sikhs and Hindus had been forcibly circumcised and their beards hacked off. The yelling of the mob came closer and closer. One day a thunderous hammering nearly splintered our door to the courtyard. "Meeeehtaaajiii! For God's sake, quick, just leave everything!" We threw open the door and there stood Sheikhji, our Muslim neighbour. "Come over to our place, quick!"

But as he spoke, a truck draw up outside and a dozen young men spilled out. Their burly leader clutched a paper from which he yelled my father's name "Devki Nandan Mehta!" Bauji nodded and the mob rushed towards our house. All my brothers and my sister and I were in the bedroom with my *Beeji*, my Mother. We huddled together in the big metal wardrobe. Beeji stood behind the door. "Stay quiet!" she hissed. We heard loud cracks and knew that shots were being fired. I was numb with fear. I saw my sister wild-eyed and shivering. Sheikhji screamed: "Devki Mehta! He is like a brother! This is a friend's house! I give you my word!" The front door slammed, the truck engine roared into life, and the house fell silent. We stayed in the dark for a long time. When Beeji finally pulled open the wardrobe door, the light streamed in and we tumbled out.

"Your family must leave!" Sheikhji said. He stayed with us until after nightfall. "Do not worry. As long as I am alive, no-one will raise a hand against you!" Under cover of dark, Kundan, our servant, silently brought the *tonga,* our two-wheeled horse-drawn carriage, to take us away. Bauji loaded his double barreled gun and slung on his cartridge belt. Beeji silently gathered together whatever she could get hold of: some food in the *tiffin* carrier, a water container and copper tumblers; some clothes and blankets in a small tin trunk. She rolled a *deri,* one of our beautiful cotton carpets, into a bedroll and tied it with silk braid she had pulled from the wall hangings.

Without a sound, we got into the tonga. Sheikhji put a sheet over our heads and we crept away into the night. "No whispering!" Beeji breathed. "Hold your breath!" she said. My younger sister Shashi and I were almost asleep when we drew into the railway station forecourt. The forecourt was in darkness save for a lone man waving a small paraffin-soaked rag on the end of a stick. But the noise and chaos of thousands of people – shaken from their beds and forced to flee with whatever they could carry – was deafening. Bewildered figures moved hither and thither in the dark, caught every now and then in the brazier's glow.

On the station platform we pushed our way through khaki-uniformed army personnel. "Quit India!" was scrawled in huge letters on every available surface. Banners held aloft read "British Out!" and "Free India!" My eldest brother Brij hoisted me up on his shoulder, my older brother Raj hurried along beside us. Bauji carried Shashi, and Beeji cradled my brother Kuckoo, our youngest, next to the tiffin-carrier. We ran towards a carriage. The army and police on the station were all Muslim and appeared very threatening. They pushed and jostled women and children and crammed them into the train carriages. Once inside the carriage, a Hindu policeman took charge. We were crammed like sardines in a tin. People spilled out of the windows and clung to the door handles.

"These are my friends! Must find room!" Sheikhji roared. We were pushed through the door and became part of a frantic, sweating, heaving crush of humanity with fear in their eyes and desperation in their voices.

"I'm not coming!" Bauji yelled above the chaos, "I'll join you later on!" and he passed Shashi through the window into the compartment. He disappeared into the crowd with Sheikhji.

Muslims gangs patrolled the station looking for Sikh and Hindu alike. They went from compartment to compartment shouting: "Sikh and Hindu out!" There were Sikhs with *kirpan* daggers very close to us, but they kept their eyes fixed ahead and did not move. I crouched on the floor with my brothers and sister. We heard yelling and screaming on the platform. Sikhs and Muslims clashed. We looked through the bars of the window and saw a body fall. Blood ran in a stream along the platform.

Kuckoo cried incessantly until he cried himself to sleep. I was in Brij's lap and he had reassuring arms around me. I could see the whites of Beeji's eyes in the flickering light of the compartment; she shook her head from side to side with terror.

Muslim police, with their large moustaches and big beards, barged into our compartment and forcibly escorted the Sikhs with their sharp and shining kirpans off the train. They threw them onto the platform. I don't know what happened to them.

One sight that lives forever in my memory is that the police on the platform told men to drop their pants to distinguish circumcised Muslims from uncircumcised Hindus. We were scared to death that the approaching policemen would demand that we drop our trousers and we wondered who was next to being taken away. The train remained in Kamalia station, while we endured the heat of an Indian August night – sweating and half crazed with fear – for what seemed an eternity

Eventually there was a huge jolt. With a shudder and a clank, the overloaded train heaved its way out of the station. We wondered if the men clinging to the outside of the train and riding on the roof would be the next to come inside our compartment and try to take us away. We were exhausted and fell asleep in spite of our cramped and desperate conditions.

I woke up to find myself curled up on the floor of the train beside my two elder brothers. A plume of smoke floated through the window. I poked my head out, and soot and coal dust flew in my eyes. I rubbed my eyes with my knuckles and made them red. Mother washed my eyes with water. "Stay away from the window!" she said. The train chugged on through the darkness. Occasionally, way over on the horizon, we passed the fierce glow of a village on fire, or the dying embers of a burnt-out temple in the fields. Many times, in the middle of nowhere, we would grind to a screeching halt, and our police escort dismounted from the train to clear the railway lines which had been blockaded by Muslims.

As the glow of dawn appeared, we stopped in the jungle. A pond glistened with dappled red early morning sun. I saw hundreds of people get down from the train and squat on the scrub land and do their morning ritual. Filling jugs and *lotkas* – copper vessels with spouts – from the pond, they washed face and hands. The smells in the close confines of our compartment became intensified with the mounting heat. The smell of food and fruit was very tempting. We were all very hungry.

"Thank God, we're out of that damn area now!" our escorting policeman exclaimed, "You can all breathe again." Mother gathered up the sheet and bedroll. She rummaged around in the string bag and produced the tiffin-carrier. "Who wants something to eat?"

"Ye-e-e-ssss! We're starving!" we all shouted. We were grimy, crumpled and bleary-eyed. We were hungry, angry, tired and filthy, our faces were streaked with soot and tears, and we still wore the clothes we had slept in. We had just endured the most horrendous night of our lives. The fifty others crammed into the carriage lay, sat and stood wherever they could. Some sat with head in hands, some stared blankly ahead, some cried. We were a trainload of shocked, bewildered and traumatised refugees. We gathered round mother and she opened the tiffin-carrier. Some families had no food with them. We shared the dried vegetable curry with other passengers nearby.

"Don't eat too much pickle, or you'll upset your stomach," Beeji whispered to me. I grinned and carried on eating my pickle. The food was not enough for all of us, but at least we had *something* to eat. There was no tea but we had water to drink from the water tank on the railway station.

"Come on, let's sit near the window!" I said.

"But we're not allowed!" said Raj.

"Aaw, come on, Beeji won't say anything. We'll see the trains coming in the opposite direction, it'll be good fun!" I whispered. I loved to feel the sudden burst of cool air on my face and, of course, hear the whistle.

In normal circumstances the trains would have thundered past each other at breakneck speed, but we were far from normal, and the long line of carriages clanked past at about thirty miles an hour. Raj and I befriended two boys whose hair was done up in a bun on the top of their heads. They were Sikh boys. We invited them to join our play. They were shy at first, but eventually they joined our "I spy with my little eye" game. My eldest brother was earnestly discussing something with Bauji. Nearby children cried upon waking, as they remembered the awful scenes they had witnessed in the night.

The train slowed to a crawl. "Get your head down!" everybody said. We pulled into a station platform. Food hawkers with baskets on their heads shouted: "Peanuts, eggs, samosas, channa, puri!" The fruit stall was set out with tangerines, mangoes and guavas. The *teawala* poured steaming milky tea into clay tumblers. The old woman sitting near us poured tea into her saucer, delicately blew on it, and then sipped it from the saucer with her eyes closed. We bought peanuts, as they were very cheap. We munched away to fill our bellies for the next few hours. We shared with our Sikh friends. As soon as the train left the platform, I shouted: "I want to pooh-pooh!"

I had never been in a train lavatory before, so I went with Brij. He helped me to get in the cubicle and I heard a roaring sound and backed off. Brij assured me it would be alright, so I took down my shorts and squatted over the hole in the cubicle floor. I was very scared as I saw the track rush by just yards below. I thought I would be sucked down through the hole and end up under the train. "I don't want to go!" I pleaded. He held me with his hand and made me sit over the hole. After I had done my business, Brij helped me to wash myself and patted my head.

When we returned to the compartment, there were smiles on the faces and a general air of relief. We caught the mood and even started to explore the compartment. "Put me on the top!" I said. Brij held out his hands so I could put my foot on each of his palms. He lifted me on his shoulder and put me on the luggage shelf high above the seats. Shashi joined me. We settled and cuddled together; talking about the food we would get at our Aunt's house. It took another three days to get to Jharia, where we would get off. Most passengers were going to the Hindu and Sikh side of the Punjab. Some had relations in Delhi, the capital, others carried on to Jaipur, and the train terminated in Calcutta. We were all homeless refugees, scattered in different directions.

What did we actually take when we made our escape? Not much. We had brought a bed sheet; a cotton carpet; the tiffin-carrier containing, dried vegetable curry, lentils and pickle; four copper tumblers; and one change of clothes for each of us; four tee-shirts, four pairs of shorts, one girl's dress, one pair of girl's knickers and a sari.

We brought no personal or legal documents and no toys – just what we wore and what we could carry.

2: Reunited

IT TOOK US FOUR DAYS and nights to get to Jharia. The journey was very difficult as the train was stopped a number of times to be checked by police or army officers. My brothers and sister and I were scared to death so we stayed quite quiet and still. Eventually we pulled slowly into Jharia Station. We had made it!

We were met by our mother's sister and brother-in-law at the station. Uncle Dina Nath and auntie Raj Kumari Kalra came hurrying down the platform, arms outstretched, to meet us.

"Thank God, Shanta, where's Devki Nandan?"

"Are the children OK?"

"We've been frantic with worry, thank God you're alright!"

Mother burst into tears. Uncle and aunt gathered us up, and, after hugs, kisses and squeezes, we left the station. Uncle hailed a tonga; we piled aboard, and set off.

Uncle Dina had a big bungalow, surrounded by a wide veranda. The verandas had glazed windows for protection from cold and monsoon downpours. The garden was extensive with a vegetable patch and an orchard full of mangoes and guava trees. There were five Kalra cousins, two sons and three daughters. Raj, the eldest, was fourteen years old. He was broad and tall. He welcomed us with a run and swirled us around. Auntie brought some *masala* tea – the family favourite – and gave it to us in copper mugs with some *barfi*, a type of cream caramel, to celebrate our safe arrival from the riots.

The town of Jharia had active coal mines. Fifty years previously there had been an explosion in a mine in the old town. The explosion caused a fire in the mine and a huge hole in the earth opened up. To that day, the fire had not been extinguished. Engineers said that sand would help stop the fire. So large quantities of it, carried by cable cars, were swung over the fire and tipped into the mine shaft. Quite often, when we lived in Jharia, we could see the night sky alive with a red glow. Sparks from the fire would fly up into the air, making me worry that we could be caught in the fire whilst asleep.

We enjoyed the company of our cousins, and played games together. Vijay was my age; we played bouncing a ball against the wall. We also jostled to pin each other down on the floor.

Our girl cousins were much older than us and they were called Pushpa, Lalita, and Sneh and they were interested in sitar-playing and singing. I was very keen on buying a yo-yo and I said to my cousin: "Let's go to the market and get one."

Vijay said: "I know a carpenter's place where they turn a piece of wood into a yo-yo." We saw the yo-yo being turned. The carpenter coloured it green and red and polished it in front of our eyes. I was better at twirling than Vijay and could make my yo-yo do anything. We played all the usual children's games: piggyback, *kanchan* (marbles on the floor), *guli danda* (a four-inch wooden ball hit by a wooden stick), hide and seek, counting the shooting stars, arm wrestling and knuckle fighting, and we watched the kite-flying

I can remember, as if it was yesterday, listening to the crackle of the radio. We listened to news of the riots very frequently, although at the time I did not realise the significance, and I certainly did not understand that we would never return to Kamalia. "This is All-India Radio. Here is the news," said the voice, "There is fighting going on in the Punjab, and Hindus are fleeing towards India. The government of India is sending trains to bring Hindus into India. Muslims are leaving for Pakistan. Leader of the Congress Party Gandhiji is touring Delhi and Calcutta in a bid to ease the tension there between Hindus and Muslims. Gandhiji has threatened to fast to death if the violence does not cease immediately."

We could hear the background noise of the crowds shouting: "Quit India!" and "Divide and Quit!" Ghandhiji broadcast an appeal: "Keep calm and bring peace in your communities!" he said. But the news was also that women and children had been slaughtered by mobs waiting in ambush for them as they escaped. Train-loads of dead and mutilated bodies reached Amritsar, the border town between India and Pakistan.

We stayed in Jharia for six months. My cousin Raj gave me the nickname *Okhi*, meaning 'boy' in Bengali, but in the Punjabi language it means 'a difficult person'. Okhi became my

15

nickname and I liked it. I felt it was affectionate, and it made everyone laugh.

Kuckoo crawled all over the floor looking for dust to put in his mouth, and then pulled a face because it was not good to eat. "Spit it out!" Beeji would say, or she would have to take it from his mouth with her fingers. This became a strange sort of joke. I can well remember eating *rasgullas*, spongy cheese balls in sugary syrup in a clay pot; it was a speciality in Bengal. Thus our young lives went on, largely unperturbed by the upheaval in our home town far away.

But, though we played, my mind was filled with worry. We knew Bauji was in danger, as he had stayed behind in Kamalia in the thick of the riots

Bauji had given up his chance to escape when he put women and children on the trucks out of Kamalia But a few months later, news came – I don't know how – that Bauji was coming out of Kamalia. He had boarded a train bound for India and lay for three days and nights clinging to the roof.

On the night we fled, after he left the station, Bauji had come upon a mob shouting: *"Pakistan jindabad, long live Pakistan!"* and *"Down with the British!"* and *"Sikhs and Hindus out!"* and *"Hindu and Sikh got too much!"* and *"Nehru sold us cheap!"* The mob was so numerous that Bauji saw no way to get to our house.

Houses and mud shacks were set alight. Amid the swirling smoke, Bauji found his way to the house of Sheikhji, our neighbour, and stayed with him. The following morning, he set off for our house, but saw from a distance that it had been set on fire in the night. Smoke still curled up from its charred remains. A part of the house remained untouched by the fire, but he saw that all the doors and windows had been smashed.

Grandfather pulled some strings. He sent a message to his brother Sirinam, to send an army truck from Delhi. The truck took two days to get to Kamalia. "Women and children and the old folks in this truck!" Bauji said, "They'll be the first out." Forty frightened souls crammed themselves into that truck and a tarpaulin was pulled up over them. They rumbled through the body-littered landscape for four days and nights. Checkpoints were heartstoppingly tense. They travelled through Lahore and reached the border city of Amritsar, the holy city for Sikhs. As soon as they crossed the border, they took off the tarpaulin. Army officers were everywhere and the truck was directed to a refugee camp for rest and refreshment. They reached Delhi in four days.

Bauji had saved forty lives. He then managed to get on to one of the last special trains to leave. The train was heaving with men frantic to go. There were not enough places in the train but no-one wanted to take the chance of staying behind. They jammed into every nook and cranny, hanging on to the train door handles and footplates. Bauji scrambled on to the roof, clinging to his rifle. He had his cartridge belt slung over his shoulder. He ducked and dived with the others on the roof, to avoid being hit through tunnels and bridges. They were covered in soot and sweat.

The train made slow progress, and screeched to a steaming halt many times as damaged and twisted railway lines, ripped apart by explosives, caused unscheduled stops. Twice they had to flee from the train as they were told that gangs of Muslims were waiting for them ahead. They decided to go into the jungle and take their chances, rejoining the train later. Two more hungry days, clinging to the roof of the train, constantly stopping in the middle of nowhere, brought them finally to an area of track so badly blown up that it was unrepairable. Now the train was going nowhere.

They were in the middle of the jungle and the train had to go back. They hacked their way through the jungle. The dense forest, although safe from the Muslim rioters, was home to many dangerous animals. They heard foxes screaming, monkeys chattering and the laughter of hyenas in the darkness of the jungle canopy. Snakes slithered across their bare feet, mosquitoes bit exposed skin, flies and ants crawled over everyone.

But the real danger came at night, when they slept on the ground. Scorpions, rats and monkeys would attack and bite any sleeping thing within reach. The refugees set up a fire and made a camp. They took it in turns to keep an eye open while others slept. They knew that rioters would be on their tail, looking for the trains they had derailed. Bauji had been a keen marksman on

17

the farm, keeping predators down with his rifle. Now he was aware that any shot would alert the Muslim rioters and give away their whereabouts. They lived on the meagre food they had and on the fruits and berries they could collect in the jungle. Two more days they stayed there.

At last, Indian army officers who were looking for them, strode into camp, gathered them up into trucks and ferried them to the station seventy miles further down the line. Bauji was bound for the east of India. The trains were sporadic and the lines were dangerous. Refugees swarmed over any available transport, like ants, completely obliterating the vehicle. They clung to anything moving either south to India for Hindus, or north to Pakistan for Muslims. He changed his journey frequently, as the way to the east had been blown up. Eventually Bauji reached Jharia. He had only his rifle on his back, and we were told about his difficult journey.

We overheard Bauji talking to Aunt Rajkumari: "The mob on the street drew closer, the sky glowed red with burning houses, we smelt the burning of flesh," he said. I later learned that the newspapers had carried pictures of murdered Hindu women and children, corpses littering the countryside. No-one cremated or buried the dead. The dogs had a feast.

Rioting, looting, burning and massacre continued all over the north. Whole trainloads of people were butchered at the stations. Many made for Jakhri, supposedly a safe haven, and six miles from Kamalia. A refugee camp was set up in Amritsar. Muslim drivers would drive no further than the border with India, and Indian drivers would not cross over into Pakistan, so change-over had to be arranged as best they could amidst the carnage and chaos. The Muslim drivers would say: "I am not going any further. I do not want to live with the sheep and pigs." Trainload after trainload of refugees fleeing across the borders was slaughtered. The dams on the rivers were opened, so anyone escaping by boat was drowned. All in all, three and a half million lives were lost.

Fazil-Ka was a border town with a Muslim majority. One night in September 1947, Muslims turned on their Hindu neighbours with such ferocity that the resultant burning set the night sky aglow for miles around. Bauji's cousin Prakash and his wife lived there. Prakash saw his wife's relations dragged out and stabbed with daggers. He said: "More than a hundred men, women and children were mutilated and slaughtered that night. The bodies were thrown into a deep pit nearby, kerosene was poured on them and they were set alight. It was hell, the screams of the dying children, no mercy, burnt alive." There is now a shrine where the pit used to be.

We were all very relieved to see Bauji safe and well. And to celebrate, my uncle and aunt arranged a picnic for us all! We travelled by truck to the picnic site, deep into the jungle near the river. The truck had an open top and the sides were painted red and green. Seats made from wooden slats ran along the back of the truck. Uncle said: "We use it to take miners to the colliery." We were very excited at the thought of riding in the truck and even more excited at the prospect of a picnic in the wild.

The journey started gently enough, but the truck gathered speed as we reached the mountain road. We could see the hills, and we started to climb up the narrow pot-holed road. The hairpin bends became more frequent. "Ooh, look! There's a big, long waterfall!" I said, as it gushed from the rock face. As we climbed higher, the truck's jerky movements made us feel sick.

"Stop the truck!" Uncle yelled. Three of us bent over the precipice and were sick. A three-hour journey brought us to our picnic spot beside a stream. We children played games. We were taken to visit an underground coalmine, as my uncle was a mining engineer.

Uncle had selected a picnic spot on a hill with a thunderous mountain stream rushing through a remote gorge into the deep valley below. My brothers and cousin were in front and I held Shashi's hand. We lagged behind with our parents. After a good hike, we returned to our picnic spot near the waterfall. Raj, Brij and my cousins Raj and Vijay swam in the stream. Beeji lowered Shashi and me down into the stream. We held on to her hand as the mountain stream swirled around us. We all felt invigorated. Bauji lay on the grass with a broad smile on his face. "I made it!" he said.

Auntie and Bauji laid out stuffed paratha omelettes, *channa* chickpeas, *dosa* rice pancakes, samosas, pasties, and spongy sweet *rasgullas* in syrup. We had a feast. But the best was yet to come. We were treated to mangoes, melon and guava. We put the water melon in a jute string bag and placed it in the stream. "Now it is cold!" Uncle declared and he sliced the melon into large red chunks, dripping with juice. Raj, Brij, Vijay and I stood by the side of the stream. "Let's skim stones on the water," I challenged Vijay. Later, we settled down for a rest and a nap.

Nightfall saw us sitting around a fire. While the elders discussed their own things, we children went off exploring the forest near the water. We sang and danced to amuse our parents. The women danced in Bengali fashion, hitting a stick in rhythm, walking a traditional Bengali dance in ring formation. Singing was provided by Pushpa and Sneh, who were good singers and sang Hindi film songs. We stayed late into the hot, humid evening. Glow-worms pulsed with their delicate light. I managed to catch some of them from the branches of a tree near the water – in fact, I had hundreds of them under my shirt and I positively glowed with their light, to the amusement of all the family. From then on, I made a point of catching glow-worms at monsoon time, and the memory delights me still.

While I was feeling safe and enjoying myself with the glow worms, special trains were being sent from Lahore to take Hindus over the border, ten to twelve thousand people to a train. Grandfather Lekhraj's brother, our grand uncle Sirinam, had fled to Delhi before the riots began. From there he had sent two trucks over the disputed border to bring out any of his relatives who could be found alive. The trucks returned bulging with grateful villagers – including Grandfather and Grandmother.

My feeling of safety among the glow worms did not last for long. Now trouble had exploded in Jharia, as the town was split down the middle. Part of the town suddenly found itself in East Pakistan, whilst the rest of the town remained in India. A mass movement, a human convoy of misery, migrated over the border to East Pakistan, which is now Bangladesh. All this chaos was compounded by the arrival in August of the monsoon rains.

Bauji's cousin Prem Lal, who lived in Delhi, gave us a single room there. Prem Lal had a small family with a daughter who was only a baby. He ran an import and export business of leather and textile goods. He was a big man with a red face and full of loud laughter. "Share with us this place until you get on your feet!" he said.

We were very pleased to go there. Being in the capital, we could get help from the government as refugees. I was in my element, running wild, catching birds and wasps and playing with my brothers and sister. We spent a few months there and none of us went to school.

But times were hard and I can well remember the food shortage. We had US military food packets called K-Rations which were sold on the black market. The rations had been floated down on India by thousands of parachutes. There were so many parachutes on the market that people made saris, blouses, skirts and curtains out of them.

There was a general shortage of cereals. America sent wheat, which was rationed – and a family ration was four pounds. One could not get *ghee*, clarified oil, on the free market, so we had to resort to the black market with its hiked prices. There was no shortage of vegetable and *daal*, the pulses which were our staple diet, but we did not eat much meat as it was too expensive. After much discussion, it was decided that we should move forty miles north, up the Grand Trunk Road, to Meerut. Mother's brother, our uncle Dharam Pal Paruthi, lived there and he had invited Bauji to start a coal delivery business with him.

This had been the greatest exodus in modern human history, east and west across the Punjab. That is how my family had to relinquish our Bauji's sixty thousand-acre farm, irrigated by the snow-fed rivers of the Himalayas, and come, cap in hand, to distant relatives. We were destitute.

3: Before the Storm

NOW I MUST TELL you some things about my family and my life before Partition.

My *Beeji*, whose maiden name was Shanta Devi, had a beautiful smiling face. I remember her dressed in her green *salwar kamiz*, Punjabi dress and trousers. She wore large dangling earrings and a small gold stud in her nose. There was a clay container from which she gave me lovely cold water.

She would tear off very small pieces of chapatti and put them in my mouth together with tiny amounts of cooked vegetable and mango. "Mare soney batey, moin kholo," she said, "My beautiful son, open your mouth."

In the afternoon we had a rest, lying on the divan. There was no electric fan, but Ramu, our servant, sat all day on the veranda, cross-legged, and pulled the rope that made the *punkha*, a large cloth hanging on bamboo canes from the ceiling, swish to and fro, thus creating a breeze. "Ramu!" mother often called, "Jaldi, jaldi punkha chalau!" Ramu would then be jolted out of his reverie and pulled the rope faster.

I was born in 1942, in Kamalia, in the Lyallpur district of the Punjab, north India. My father, Devki Nandan, had two brothers, Bodhraj and Hari Krishan. Uncle Hari Krishan lived next door to us. Our houses were identical. They were built of handmade bricks with mud and cow dung floors. The flat roof was made from supporting planks of wood, across which was placed straw, then round flat tiles of hardened cow dung and finally a coating of raw sugar known as *jaggery,* to make it watertight. We had verandas on all sides. Our house had eight large rooms. We had a large courtyard and walls covered with flowery plants, which looked very tall to me as a five-year-old.

My Bauji and my Beeji came from families that had farmed in Kamalia for generations. There were five children including me in our family, the others were my older brothers, Brij and Raj, my younger brother Krishan (always known as Kuckoo) and my little sister Shashi.

The afternoons were very enjoyable, as we three boys played games on the divan before eventually falling asleep. We played *carrom*, an eastern version of tiddly-winks, or we got out the snakes and ladders or playing cards."

"C'mon hurry up!" Raj hissed in the hopes that we would make a mistake and lose the game. Brij never succumbed to Raj's tactics but remained his usual unflappable and calm self. Brij, tall slim and elegant, was our beloved eldest brother whom we admired. Raj and I, all scabby knees and untidy hair, wore faded tee-shirts and short trousers; Kuckoo was a baby, a few months old. He lay, totally naked, in his wooden cot. Sarjoni, a servant girl, often settled on the floor beside the cot to rock him off to sleep.

Shashi was two years younger than me. She stayed with Beeji, watching her knitting, or playing pat-a-cake with Sarjoni. Shashi was always smiling. I remember her, darting here and there, quick and nimble as a little butterfly in her brightly coloured dress.

The courtyard walls glowed terracotta red in the afternoon sunshine. Mauve bougainvilia flowers climbed all over the walls and threw deep shadows on the courtyard compound. I loved being in the shadows because the sun was so fierce. Bees buzzed around the sacred basil plants that grew in the copper pots on the veranda. Sarjoni's ankle bracelets jingled as she busied herself with household chores around the courtyard.

My earliest memory of my father is my running out of the courtyard shouting: "Bauji! Bauji!" when I heard horse's hoofs in the road. I knew it was Raja, our horse, bringing Bauji home. He dismounted, scooped me up and flung me high in the air, then caught me and gave a huge hug and squeeze. He appeared a very tall man as he lifted me up on his shoulders.

He was dressed in a fine white cotton *salwar,* the Punjabi trouser, and a loose shirt, the *kamiz,* which flowed behind him in the breeze. He wore a white turban wrapped around his head which was fashioned in the Punjabi way, with a proud stiffened fan shape that stood to one side of his head. He wore pointed leather riding boots. He sat me on the horse, which he had been riding all day at the farm, and we trotted around the courtyard together. Raja, the white and brown horse, seemed very tall. He chewed on the bit and stamped the earth. I loved the multi-coloured plumes on his head, fluttering in the air. I watched Kundan the servant cut fodder for Raja in a hand-driven cutting machine.

The house was outside Kamalia town, near the railway line. We could hear the trains clearly from our house, and I would run around, screeching, hissing and whistling like an engine in the shunting yard. We were brought up with clanking engines steaming past our house day and night. We would line up, one behind the other, Brij at the front and me bringing up the rear, as we hissed and tooted our way along the road. We would hear the sound of an approaching engine and send Raj to ask Bauji if we could go and see it. We joined in. "Please, Bauji, we want to go to see the engine." Bauji accompanied us as we stood on the platform. The biggest, blackest engine roared in through a cloud of steam, hissing loudly as its wheels screeched to a halt. We were thrilled.

There was an inter-connecting door between the courtyard of our house and the house of my uncle Hari Krishan, and we often played with our cousins. Sushma, Ashok and Narinder would burst through the courtyard door at any time of the day, and – with a "Come on, let's fly kites!" – we were off to play.

Sushma, being a girl, would skip in to see Shashi and they played together often. Ashok and Narinder, the sons of the family, sought out us boys and we spent our early years in and out of each other's houses. Ashok was my age and we would scamper around the courtyard, trying to catch a flapping minah bird or scurrying squirrel. Narinder was the age of my elder brother Raj. Narinder's nickname was Nano. "Nano, Nano! Give me a piggyback!" I would shout, and Nano would hoist me up on his back and away we would go around the compound and out on the road. Raj and Narinder seemed to be always testing their strength against each other with endless arm wrestling and bare knuckle fights. "Come on, you can beat him!" I shouted to Raj.

Chuhamal, my great grandfather inherited 240,000 acres of prime farmland in the Punjab, watered by the five mighty rivers running from the Himalayas. The word *Punjab* means Land of Five Rivers. He divided the land equally, giving 60,000 acres to each of his four sons, one of whom was my Grandfather Lekhraj.

Grandfather Lekhraj lived in an enormous farmhouse with thirty- one rooms, eighteen downstairs and thirteen upstairs. He married Parvati-Devi, a renowned beauty in her day who, out of modesty, kept her head covered at all times

Kumar Sen is an area of sixty square miles in the district of Lyallpur, which is now called Faislabad, in Pakistan. The Maharajah of Kumar Sen was under-age, and Lekhraj was given executive powers over four towns in the area. He held a court regularly and was fond of sending for his grandson Brij to come and sit with him. Brij was carried on a sedan chair by servants, never walking any distance at all, until he was five years old.

As a reward for his services to the State, grandfather was given eight villages. He sank the first artesian well in the whole of the province and bought the first motor car in the area –a Morris Minor. A man before his time, his last will and testament ensured his daughter inherited the same as his sons. He divided his 60,000-acre estate into six equal shares, one each for himself, his wife and his four children.

The privileged surname *Mehta* was bestowed on him by the Maharajah. Mehta is a title that means *head of the village* or *landlord.*

My mother first saw my father at the *Mohurram Fair* as he came riding towards her on a white horse. Mother's mother was dead, so she was cared for by her elder sister.

She said: "The boy on the white horse is the right one for me."

Her sister said: "If you like him, a match can be made."

The two exchanged glances but there was no conversation at all, as it was not a tradition to talk to your future husband! They married when she was 17 years old.

4: Bitten!

"AAAAAAAGHHH!! IT BIT ME! Aaaah! Ma-maaaa!" Dark red blood welled up from the puncture marks in my arm. It dropped in big shiny spheres onto the dusty road and shimmered there a moment in the sunlight, before melting away into the ground.

A dog, so thin its bones almost stuck through its sandy coloured coat, bounded along beside me. Saliva hung in strands from the foam around its mouth. It yelped and nibbled at bald patches and scabs on its back. Maybe I patted it, but most likely I pulled its tail. Whichever it was, it swung round and sank its yellow teeth into my flesh, all the while growling and shaking its head vigorously from side to side, wrenching my arm in its socket.

I stood in the middle of the road and yelled. I was five years old.

Beeji ran towards me, squeezed my arm until more blood oozed out and rolled her handkerchief over the wound. Brij, my elder brother, came puffing up, hitting the dog with stones and ran after it. It ran away on three legs and disappeared into the bazaar. Beeji quickly shouted for a *rikshawala* and lifted me in her lap, jumped into rikshaw and told the rikshawala to go fast. We turned towards home.

To distract me from screaming, the rikshawala said: "Look at the plumes on the horse's head on that tonga on the road." The plumes were ruffling and shimmering in the sunshine, but that did not amuse me. We reached home and Beeji cleaned and dressed the wound.

In spite of her care, the wound quickly became very painful and inflamed. Dr. Chopra was sent for and he listened as mother described the dog. He uncovered my arm and examined the teeth marks with a frown. He looked very grave and said: "You need to find the dog in the next twenty four hours. If you can't, we'll have to assume the dog has rabies. We can't wait and see, Mrs Mehta, rabies kills!"

He went on: "Unless you find the dog and we see that it's fit and healthy, I'm sending little Sat here for an emergency course of anti-Rabies treatment. You'll have to go to Delhi for that." We were stunned.

The family searched all over town to find the dog, but without success. "We will kill the dog!" they told me.

I went to Delhi, fifty miles away, by train. It took us three hours. I spent the first half of the journey sobbing. I shed tears all over my Beeji and then fell asleep in her lap. We went to stay with my uncle Dewan and auntie Janak. Uncle was an engineer in the army and auntie, my father's sister, a real beauty, suffered from very delicate health. They had a *kothi*, a large house with a huge garden and had servants and a driver provided by the army.

I enjoyed the excitement and novelty of going to hospital, until it became clear that I was to have fourteen anti-rabies injections. The doctor said "We've got to presume the dog is infected with rabies, so we've no alternative but to go ahead with the treatment."

Then, turning to me, he said: "Better safe than sorry, eh, sonny?" I was taken to the hospital every day for two weeks and given an injection in my abdomen with what looked like a *huge* needle,

The following day I slipped out of Beeji's grasp "I don't want it! I don't want it!" I shouted over my shoulder as I ran out of the door and away down the corridor. Uncle pelted after me and swept me up in his arms. I kicked and shouted at the top of my voice. In the end, they got hold of my arms and legs.

"Grit your teeth boy and be brave!" my uncle roared, "It won't hurt!" It certainly *did*. Beeji was extremely upset and tears ran down her face. "Will my son be alright?" she repeatedly asked the doctor. As a small child, I could not imagine how injections in my tummy would help.

I soon regained my usual form and began again exploring my world. I spent most of my time looking into every part of my uncle's kothi. The garden had wonderful fruit trees, and I would climb the trees and pick the fruit to my heart's content. There were ten-foot-tall guava trees, with their fragrant greenish-yellow fruits. As I climbed, a number of bright green and red parrots would shoot out of the branches, leaving behind their half-nibbled meals. Uncle also had a mango orchard. The trees were twenty-five foot giants. I would climb high into the branches, and disappear in the shiny, broad-leaved foliage. The fruits were small, hard and green, ripening into large golden-yellow globes. I sat on my perch and squeezed the juice out until it dripped off my chin and down my arms. *Bair* bushes were easy to raid, and I could nip one or two of the sweet-and-sour fruits off as I passed by. "Come down from that tree immediately, Sat!" I could hear mother as she shouted from the doorway. I did *not* come down!

The guava trees were home to a number of hornets' nests. I was unafraid of the hornets, and I often watched them as they went about their activities. I caught a large black and yellow hornet with a towel. I put the towel over the hornet but to my surprise, I found there was more than one. Several came out of the towel and flew at my face and hands. I screamed at the top of my voice and tried to get rid of them. I ran towards the house screaming: "Beeji! Beeji!"

She came running towards me and took me into the house. She wrung a cloth under the cold water pump and slapped it to my forehead. "How many times have I told you not to play with wasps? You put grey hairs on my head!" I had a very bad reaction to the stings: my eye, then my entire face, became very swollen, and I had great difficulty in opening my eyes. I was rushed to hospital and had to have more injections. I was kept in overnight.

As I sat in the hospital bed, half blind and unable to talk, I was very, very scared. Mother stayed with me all night. In the early hours of the morning, I started having difficulty breathing. "I am going to die!" I thought, and had to have another injection.

Later that day, my face swelling began to subside and I was discharged from the hospital. Beeji and I stayed with my uncle and aunt a few more days, so that the swelling could go down further. The hornet left on my forehead two scars which I carry to this day, and they are my personal reminder of the day the insect world decided to teach me a lesson.

5: Historical Meerut

AFTER OUR TERRIBLE EXODUS, we moved to Meerut, about eighty kilometres north of Delhi, on the Grand Trunk Road to Dehradun.

The seeds of The First War of Independence were sown in Meerut Military Cantonment when, in the summer of 1857, resentment with the occupying British forces became a revolt. It was said that practices highly offensive to the religious beliefs of Indian soldiers had been employed in the manufacture and maintenance of British issue ammunition. At that time it was necessary to bite the end off the gun cartridges and it was said that the cartridges had been greased with pork fat. This is offensive to Muslims because the pig is considered unclean.

Furthermore, it was said that the guns were greased with fat from the cow, an animal sacred to Hindus. I believe this is true, as it was explained to us in school and in the history books. The uprising spread from Meerut to Delhi and Kanpur. The Kali Paltan, beside Sadar Bazaar, in Meerut Cantonment, is the spot where the very first shot was fired. The temple commemorates those Founder Members of the Independence Movement who died there in 1857

As schoolchildren, we visited the temple and were proud of our heritage and the stand that our forefathers had made in the pursuit of freedom for us. We took our shoes off at the gate, washed our hands, and then gathered some marigold flowers as an offering. As we entered the temple, we struck the big bell. We knelt before the statue of god Shiva and then collected our *prasad* (gifts from the temple altar).The temple garden was set out in typical Hindu style. It had a huge shady *peepul* tree under which the worshippers gathered. The branches appeared to connect two worlds.

We took holy water in our cupped hands, touched our lips and then threw the water over our head. The holy water was fragrant with *tulsi,* Indian basil herb. Banana and jasmine also grew there, the fruits and flowers of which were used in religious worship. Red-faced, long-tailed monkeys swung high in the branches of the *peepul* tree. Monkeys also played on the wall surrounding the temple compound, next to the vendors selling peanuts and fruits. I loved the strangely compelling music played by a band of stick-thin men seated in the dust outside the temple compound. They were dressed in clothes from the Rajasthan region and when they smiled they all had gold teeth. As we wandered in the shady temple garden, under the trees, we tried to understand India's ninety-year struggle for Independence.

In early childhood I was intrigued by the men called eunuchs. They came from an area of Meerut which was predominantly Muslim. Some befriended me because many of my Bauji's employees came from the area where they lived. They would tell me jokes, make funny faces and dance to the assembled people on the road. I was never scared of them, but could not work out whether they were men or women.

They would speak with a man's voice but dress and behave like a woman, wearing very brightly coloured clothes and dangling jewellery. They wore their hair long and had very red lips. They would mince along the road, dancing and clapping their hands, making a lot of noise and asking if there were any celebrations nearby, such as weddings or births. They would arrive, uninvited, at wedding receptions two or three days before the ceremony and keep the large numbers of guests entertained, dancing and singing, accompanied by hand-clapping and much audience participation. At the conclusion of the ceremonies, the eunuchs received food and money. The family members held money in their hands, making circular movements around the heads of the eunuchs. Eunuchs are supposed to bring good luck.

Then, with much head-tossing and swirling of skirts, and more noisy singing and hand-clapping, the eunuchs would take their leave, blessing the family and, depending on the ceremony, praying for a successful marriage or happiness with the new baby.

My friend Kamlesh said: "They are neither male nor female; they cannot have babies, which means they are impotent." He went on: "They live on the fringes of society, earning a living by singing and dancing at parties, prostitution and begging." It sounded to me as if Kamlesh had been to the library.

We moved from our home in Delhi to Meerut in the spring of 1948. We found a place to live, in the Tehsil district of Meerut. It was the poorest area, inhabited mostly by Muslims.

We were a Hindu family, but we had nowhere else to go. We rented three rooms on the first floor of a dilapidated and crumbling building in a dark and narrow street. The building was structurally unsound and in a bad state of repair. But Beeji set about making it as homely as she could for us. We tripped and stumbled over uneven floors, crumbling brickwork and leaking pipes. Mother became increasing anxious for our safety and constantly reminded us to *be careful and don't run!* It was very cold and felt unsafe. The house was such that we could feel the monsoon coming through the wall, green and black mould spread slimy fingers in the corners of the rooms. But because of our financial situation, it was the only house we could afford to rent. Neighbours said the house brought nothing but bad luck to anyone who lived there. We even heard it whispered that the house was haunted. We belong to a sect of Hinduism known as Arya Samaj – and, as such, did not believe in ghosts, devils, ghouls or witches.

In the evenings we put kerosene oil lamps all around the house. In the alcove, Beeji placed a *deva*, a small clay pot containing oil and a wick. But the deva would not stay alight. She gradually began to suspect that the neighbours were right, and that the house was haunted with evil spirits which, amongst other mishaps, also extinguished the light in the alcove. On occasions we would hear thumping sounds in the night as if somebody was walking on the roof. We began to be scared. Bauji reassured us it was only a cat on the rooftop.

In spite of our previous disregard for ghosts, we experienced a catalogue of bad luck in the house. It all began as the monsoon season started. There had been a heavy downpour for a number of days and the rain came through the roof. One day we heard a loud creaking and then a crash. Bauji went to check the courtyard and, as he did so, the floor gave way and he disappeared through the floor and landed on the ground beneath, in a heap of tumbling rubble. Beeji came rushing through, wondering what the boys were up to now. She also fell through the hole and landed on top of Bauji. Luckily, both had only a few cuts and bruises. Within days of that, my little brother Kuckoo fell over and broke his collar bone. The candles in the house still would not stay alight, and bad luck continued to dog our family.

We could now feel the presence of the ghost and we were convinced that it was a lady whose spirit had not come to rest. Mother wrung her hands and screamed: "Go away! You've caused nothing but misery to my family! You're the cause of our bad luck!" Often we would hear the wooden *charpoy* bed being tossed into the air and landing with a loud crash on the flat roof upstairs. The evil presence would then go to the kitchen and violently rattle the pans hanging from nails on the wall.

One day, as we gathered on the floor to eat, Beeji appeared in the doorway, ashen-faced and clearly very upset. Her voice was shaking as she said: "Something has just tried to pull the storm lamp out of my hands. I felt a tug, and someone tried to snatch the lamp, but I managed to hold on to it!" She was frightened by the aggressiveness of the incident. She was at her wits' end with the increasingly sinister atmosphere of the house and the violent and threatening behaviour of our aggressive guest. She was of a very practical and down-to-earth nature and furthermore was not overly religious. However, she decided to ask for outside help.

She set off immediately and walked to the Hindu temple. There she begged for God's blessing. When she returned, she set up an area in one corner of the room as a little altar for prayers. There, every morning and evening, we gathered to light little deva lamps and burn incense sticks and placed these on a copper plate, on which she then traced a circular motion before the altar whilst saying the *Gayatri* prayer. She completed the ceremony by dipping her finger in vermilion paste and touching it to each of her children's foreheads. She then pressed a few grains of rice on the red mark on our foreheads to ward off evil and she and Bauji then turned to each other and placed the mark on each other's forehead. The ceremonies did not change anything and the bad luck continued.

Beeji arranged for a *pundit* – a Hindu priest – to come over from the temple to dispel the evil spirits. To make doubly sure, she also invited the *muezzin* from the Muslim Masjid nearby! We as a family prayed for help and lived from day to day.

6: Broken Wing

IT WAS HIGH SUMMER and the temperature across India climbed into the forties. Meerut, on the Deccan plateau, was hot and dry, like walking into a hot oven.

"Crushed ice, flavoured ices, iiice, and iiice!" The ice-cart man had come. He was in the alleyway with a big block of dripping ice on his cart. I had to find some money and get to him quick before he went away. It was the summer that I was eight years old. I grabbed a penny from mother's shelf and skipped down the concrete steps, taking them two at a time to the alleyway. My feet slipped from under me and I went tumbling down, head over heels. I came to a stop at the bottom of the steps, looking up at the sky. I could feel the penny but was unable to open my hand to see it. I was unable to move at all to begin with, so I lay there looking at the sky. I eventually tried to get up and go in search of the ice-man. My legs could move, but when I looked at my upper half, the left arm was torn and bleeding and my elbow bone poked out like a big white icicle, through the skin. I screamed at the top of my voice and then passed out.

When I came round, Bauji was carrying me upstairs in his arms. I felt very scared and clung on for reassurance. I thought this would stop all my games and activities for a while. We took a three-wheeler rickshaw to the local Municipal Hospital. There were crowds of people in the casualty area, all with plasters and dressings. Nurses were running frantically to and fro. The casualty doctor lifted the cloth in which mother had wrapped my elbow. He hastily replaced it when he saw the jagged sharp end of bone, and a black blood clot – the size of a man's fist – slithered to the floor.

He called the senior doctor, Dr Gandhi, from his outpatient clinic to come over urgently to see me. Dr Gandhi examined my elbow again. The two doctors withdrew to a corner, heads together, and discussed how best to treat me. Looking very grave, they eventually came across to Bauji and drew him aside. I was all ears and overheard the words: "Operation…outcome, not sure… save arm…." Bauji glanced over to me. Blood had soaked through the cloth and now plopped in great red drops on the examination couch. I was holding on to a nurse with my good arm and I was sobbing. I saw stars before my eyes and felt very faint and weak. The nurse tried to take away my brother's torn shirt dressing. It was soaked in blood and had become stuck to my elbow. I screamed my head off and started shouting: "Don't you touch it, don't touch it!"

After a great deal of persuasion, I let my sobs die down. I gritted my teeth as the nurse cleaned my deformed elbow, swabbing round the bone and washing away the blood. But I was in agony and could not stop kicking and screaming. The nurse put on a new dressing and a splint. "We will soon put it right. Let us get you to the ward," she said. I was still waving my good hand and shouting when I was put on a trolley and rushed to the ward.

There were very strong smells of curry, sweat and ammonia in the corridor. I was wheeled into the ward and could see everybody looking towards me. As the children's ward was full and I was an emergency admission, I had to be in the adult ward. This ward was full of people crying, sniffling, moaning and sighing. It was a terrible place of misery. I wanted to scream and run away. I started crying uncontrollably. I then got violent hiccups. I was very scared and I could feel thumping noises in my ears and chest. My throat was sore with crying and my eyes were stinging with sweat. After a while I took stock of my surroundings. The ward was a long room with beds on both sides. There were two or three mobile screens of dirty green cloth placed around the beds of patients who were either using a bedpan or dying.

I went to the operating theatre the same afternoon. I was asked to breathe through a mask as a doctor poured drops of liquid on it. They asked me to count. "One, two, three, and four…" I could smell something strong from the mask, so I started fighting it and wanted to jump off the table. They got hold of me, and all I remember after that is counting up to ten or eleven. I woke up in a hospital bed with the strong smell still in my nostrils, and a thumping headache.

"I feel sick," I said.

"Suck some ice cubes," said mother.

I had a huge, heavy, damp plaster on my arm. The next day I had recovered reasonably well from the anaesthetic and started walking around the ward. The next few days I spent in the hospital garden, watching kites flying high in the sky.

A large yellow kite with red borders swept over the hospital garden. The sound of flapping paper wings, dipping and sweeping over my head, was the first familiar and comforting thing that had happened to me since I had come into the hospital.

There must have been another dozen kites in the sky. There were boys putting out their *manjha*, a glass-covered thread on spools. They licked their fingers and held them up in the air to check the wind. Some kites were rolled from side to side. The breeze wafted through my hair and the wind was perfect for flying. There were children running around on the hospital lawn, playing with a ball. I felt free and happy. My mind drifted upwards with the kite and I wished myself away from this place, floating away into the clouds like the kite.

As I had a fracture and the bone had come through the skin, I was prescribed penicillin injections. Bauji had to find the money to buy the very expensive penicillin. He also had to be very sure the drug was pure. There were many worthless imitation medicines on the market, so Bauji sought out a pharmacist he knew and trusted.

Bauji was of a very peaceful nature, seldom known to raise his voice in anger. But on this occasion he yelled at Beeji and me: "You can't have penicillin from just any old chemist. They'll sell milk done up in phials, looks just the same. Liars! They don't care!"

He went on: "We've got to get the right stuff; infection in the bone can kill you. Corrupt, lying chemists shouldn't be trusted to cure even a dog!" It was clear Bauji was at the end of his endurance.

We got the genuine penicillin, but it had to be stored at a constant cool temperature, and so we borrowed a thermos flask from somewhere, in which to keep my life-saver. I had an injection every four hours for the next two months. The injections were given in my bottom with a large needle and glass syringe. It was then put in a sterilizer and boiled up to be re-used repeatedly. I was constantly anxious, thinking of the next one, and it was compounded by the pain and discomfort from the operation site and the itchy and irritating plaster. I had a sore bottom on both sides and one day I did ask Father: "Will I have holes in my bottom with all these injections?" My brothers and friends, visiting, teased me, calling me "Sat Sore Bum."

This was a very sad time for me and I cried frequently. As I looked at my arm, I thought: *I am never going to come out of hospital.* In the end I was discharged from the hospital after a two-month stay. When I got home, I set to work building up the tone of the muscles of my arm, holding a piece of rock salt a kilo in weight. I did my exercises in the courtyard in the sun. I could feel the rock salt melting in my hand. I had to squeeze my fingers on the rock until my forearm muscles tightened and I could see them move. To improve my shoulder strength, I lifted my plastered arm towards the sky. I circled my arm round and round, and daily my strength grew. I had lots of *Get well* messages written by nurses, friends, brothers and sister. When I felt mischievous, I used my plastered arm as a weapon to thump my brothers and school friends.

My plastered arm was very itchy and I often scratched down inside the plaster cast with knitting needles or wooden sticks. My parents and the nurses warned me repeatedly that if I kept scratching with needles, I would introduce infection and the fracture wound would not heal. But I thought that, as the plaster was getting slightly loose, it would help to get air under the plaster and that would heal my arm faster. One day, a few fat white grubs came crawling from the top of my plaster. I frantically shook my arm and they dropped to the floor. I stamped on them. They were maggots and I remembered a fly had crawled out from under my plaster a while before. She had laid her eggs in my wound! Bauji looked very concerned. "I'll take you to Dr Chopra straight away. He'll clean your arm!"

Dr. Chopra examined my elbow and plaster very carefully. I cried: "My arm has gone rotten and maggots are eating it." But he said: "These grubs get rid of dead tissue and clean up the area."

I did not find that reassuring. I was worried to death. I attended the hospital three months later and my plaster was removed. Despite a full course of penicillin, I had developed an infection of the bone causing foul white liquid to pour out of the wound. I was very despondent, but continued with my elbow exercises and building up the muscles in my arm. I was used to exercising; but now the plaster was off, I felt free to swing my arm. I would put a pound weight of rock salt in my hand and lift my arm to shoulder height. The movement and muscle strength began to build up. I would let my arm swing down so it became straight.

I exercised away from the public gaze. I was aware of my deformed arm and wore a long-sleeved shirt so nobody would see it. In the hot sun, the rock salt melted and irritated the skin of my arm. We were told that my injury would improve with time, but I was still very upset and used to look at my elbow in the mirror and cry. It restricted my adventurous spirit and I was getting behind with my schooling. I was seen a few times at the municipal hospital and could hear murmurs about amputation if the infection were not controlled. Bauji and Beeji consoled me and did their best to seek advice.

Bauji wrote to my uncles and aunts and explained my situation. He asked if they knew of any specialist who could help. Dr Chopra, our family doctor, was very helpful and was definitely against amputation. He advised us to seek advice in Delhi Hospital. There was talk about a tuberculous infection affecting my elbow, as the white stuff continued pouring out and the wound refused to heal.

We were introduced through Father's third cousin to a bone specialist: Colonel Santok Singh, an army colonel in Meerut Cantonment. Col Singh sent an army jeep and his driver to collect us and take us to see him at his *kothi*, set in extensive gardens within the cantonment. Colonel Singh was a very large man, bald-headed but with a lovely big moustache, which he had rolled and waxed at the sides. He always dressed in a khaki uniform.

I was scared to death, my heart jumping all over the place, as I thought he might advise an amputation. We spent over two hours at the house, where we had tea and biscuits. His advice in the end, delivered in his deep booming voice, was a huge relief. In his opinion I should have a further course of penicillin injections. He said that in the army he had seen many such wounds and they usually healed. But he went on to say that if the penicillin did not clear the infection, there would be nothing to be gained from further surgery, except amputation.

Bauji asked all our relatives for help regarding my arm infection, trying to avoid amputation at any cost. My uncle Jai Nath Dewan, thought of a way to help. His brother was in the Ministry of Health and had told uncle that there was a world famous orthopaedic Professor visiting Delhi who might help me.

Flying with a Broken Wingegment>

7: The Professor

I WAS TAKEN TO IRWIN HOSPITAL in Delhi and was seen in the outpatient department by Professor Robert Roaf from Liverpool, England. Professor Roaf was on sabbatical leave to work in India for a few months.

When my name was called, Bauji and I went into the Professor's consulting room. There were about six other doctors in the room. He stood up and extended his hand across the desk to Bauji and me in a firm handshake. I found this very reassuring. He was over six feet tall and looked young for a professor. He had blond hair, with a parting in the middle. He had rosy cheeks and bushy eyebrows. He was always smiling. He would have a good laugh at anything amusing and he made the people around him relax. The doctors watched as he examined me. He explained that "a serious bone infection and mal-union of a compound fracture has led to marked restricted mobility of the elbow."

He said: "It may be possible to get rid of the bone infection. Then we can look at the elbow function." He stressed that there was no guarantee and there would be some remaining deformity.

I nudged Bauji and murmured: "I want to ask a question."

Professor Roaf noticed my agitation. "What is worrying you, little chap?"

I blurted out: "Are you going to cut my arm off?"
He gave me a wink and a smile. "You'll keep your arm! We'll get rid of the infection. And then we'll repair the fracture."

The clinic was very busy with the waiting room full of people. There were patients encased in a full body plaster from neck to ankle who had tuberculous deformity of the spine. I later learned that Professor Roaf was a world leader in the treatment of tuberculous deformity and had pioneered new surgical procedures for such cases. Indian specialists sent their worst cases of bone infection and mal-aligned fractures to see the Professor. "Send me your hopeless cases!" he said.

A few weeks later I was admitted to Irwin Hospital. As I had already spent ten weeks in Meerut Hospital, the prospect of

40

more hospital held no fears. And I had been assured by Professor Roaf himself that I would keep my arm. I thought: *There is a God in this world and He has sent somebody to make me better.*

Even so, I had learned to be modest in my hopes. I still wondered at times if I would return home with or without my arm. I had a bone infection, medically named osteomyelitis; I had undergone three unsuccessful operations, and endured courses of painful injections of dubious penicillin. All this made me mature and I was able to ask Bauji about the possibility of an amputation and how life would be without my arm. They were very straight and said: "We will do everything possible on this earth and leave no stone unturned to get you better. You are a very lucky boy to have an operation by such a special surgeon from England. The Professor will do his best to save your arm and make your elbow work properly."

Irwin Hospital was a big sprawling building with huge corridors. I saw first-hand the procedures and daily running of a big Delhi hospital. The day after my admission, Professor Roaf was on his ward rounds with other doctors and nursing staff. Professor Roaf had six Indian doctors, all specializing in bone surgery, accompanying him. There was also an English nursing sister, an Indian matron, other nursing staff and physiotherapists.

The Indian doctors admired Professor Roaf and were very keen to learn from his expertise. The pace of the round was slow. There was much discussion amongst the surgeons. My turn came, and the entourage arrived and surrounded my bed. The Professor greeted me with a smile and said: "How is this young man today?" I could understand that amount of English as I had been learning and practising English during my wait to be admitted.

They examined my elbow; they checked the movement and prodded the infected sore on the front of my elbow. After discussion, Professor Roaf said: "You will have your operation tomorrow."

On the ward round was Sister Margaret, the English nursing sister accompanying Professor Roaf; and I confided to her my concern about the loss of my arm. When the entourage came to my bed, Sister Margaret was smiling and held my right hand while the doctors examined my elbow. The Prof and other surgeons stood above my bed and discussed my surgery. I became more and more agitated and upset, tears started flowing down my cheeks, and I shouted, in English: "Amputation!" I made a gesture as if to chop my arm off.

Immediately Sister Margaret said: "No, no!" She put her arms around me and wiped away my tears with a piece of cotton gauze. I said to Bauji, in Hindi, that I was very scared. Bauji translated into English to Sister Margaret. She said: "Brave boy, don't cry, and don't worry. I will be with you in the operating theatre tomorrow."

Sister Margaret was a very tall lady in her thirties. She had mid-length blonde hair and blue eyes and a perfectly straight nose. She had rosy cheeks and wore bright red lipstick. As she passed by, a lovely whiff of perfume lingered in the air after her. She wore a blue dress and a full and flowing triangular starched white cap. She said: "The Professor has treated many patients like you in England. They have all been successful. You will be alright." She was very friendly, and asked me to teach her Hindi while she taught me more English.

This friendship flourished over my eight weeks in the hospital, and we both kept our promises. She was interested in Hindi words meaning *thank you, please, love you, good morning, goodbye,* and *how are you?* Sister Margaret on the ward tried to communicate with patients in Hindi. We would rehearse her Hindi when she came to see me. We tried some of the common sentences. She became good at Hindi and could speak about ten sentences, but with an English accent.

As soon she walked near me, she would say: "Aap ka kia hall hay?" ("How are you?")

I replied "Mein theek thak hoin." ("I am alright.")
I would ask her: "Aapka shubh naam kya hai?" ("What is your name?")

Sister replied: "Mera naam Margaret hai."

We tried other useful sentences: "Darvasa band kauro" ("Close the door") and "Punkha chalau" ("Put on the fan"). She asked me especially to teach her the following sentences: *Kya aap Angrezi samajhte hain?* (Do you understand English?); *Chithi lejao aur jawab lao* (Take the message and bring back the answer); *Jeldi jeldi chalau* (Walk fast, fast!); *Ham sat baje guram gusal maimgte hain* (I would like to have a bath at 7 o'clock); and *Barash ho reehi hai* (It is raining).

The day before my operation, preparations were made. My elbow was thoroughly washed with antiseptic, painted with yellow solution, and covered completely by bandages. On the morning of my surgery, I was very hungry but there was a hand-written notice on my bed number which read: *No Drinks or Food.*

"It's not fair! I've been fasting since last night and not had a drink. I should get some drink at least," I whined.

"Stop it!" said the Indian Sister, "you won't get your operation if you eat or drink."

I was taken to the operating theatre but I was not frightened. I just wanted to get better. In the anaesthetic room a mask was placed on my face and once again I was asked to count. This time, by holding my breath, I reached 16; had I not done so, I would have been asleep by ten.

The next thing I remember is coming round in the ward, whilst Bauji gave me ice cubes to stop my retching and vomiting. This anaesthetic was just as bad as the one at the other hospital. My plaster was wet and very heavy, but it soon dried.

Next morning I was on my feet exploring the ward. Sister said I would have breakfast of double *roti* (toast in hot milk) which was a rare treat. Very soon, I could be found exploring the hospital garden, watching kites. In the evening, Bauji came bearing a bag of fruit.

My condition over the next few days improved and I got used to being in the hospital. As the only child in the ward and in spite of being in plaster, I was given small tasks like taking notes and things for the doctors and nurses, gradually learning a lot about other patients' problems.

With the encouragement of Sister Margaret, I was allowed to walk with the Professor and his entourage and be part of the ward round, an experience which would affect my whole future. I had a bed next to the nurse's station. The adult patients did not seem to mind me. If they needed something fetching, I was always there.

I could walk all over the hospital grounds and beyond, outside the gates and on the streets if I wanted to. I made myself useful in explaining and reassuring some patients who did not know the ward procedure. Or I spent time chatting with patients who were not visited by any relatives or friends. The ward was full of very ill people: there were tuberculous cold abscesses of the spine, and polio-affected adults with deformities. There were young men paralysed from motorbike accidents, and patients with raised legs on traction.

After four weeks I was told they needed to change the plaster for a lighter one – again, a quick anaesthetic and the plaster was changed. During the next few weeks in hospital, I had physiotherapy in the form of hand and arm exercises which, I was told, were very important. The arm exercises had become second nature to me – I had been doing them for such a long time. Bauji brought some small weights from a fruit and vegetable shop in the market and I started lifting these. I used particularly to hang down the weights in the hopes that my arm would eventually become straight.

The night staff were good to me; they even knitted for me a sleeveless jumper which I treasured. The jumper was hand-knitted from dark blue Cashmere wool. It had a band of red around the neck. It was very cozy and kept me warm. I loved wearing it and every time I wore it, I thought of the kind staff nurse from Tamil Nadu who had made it for me. When I had grown out of it, I passed it on to my younger brother Kuckoo. He wore it until it fell to pieces.

My plaster was very, very itchy, the hot climate particularly caused it to sweat and I often got into trouble from the ward sister, particularly at night, for borrowing her knitting needle to put down the plaster and give my arm a good scratch.

"Stop it! You are at it again! No wonder your family calls you *Okhi*! Difficult! You are the most naughty, difficult child I have ever come across."

During the day I would venture into the hospital corridors and got a good feel for the work that took place, getting quite upset sometimes at seeing people very ill and in pain. I saw first-hand the procedures and daily running of a big Delhi hospital. I was the only child Professor Roaf treated during the eight weeks I spent at Irwin Hospital. I was also the only child on the orthopaedic adult ward.

There was a pattern to the ward routine: a flurry of activity in the morning before the ward round. There were patients being collected for the operating theatre and other patients returning from it. There were porters and nurses with masks hanging round their necks. There was a midday hustle with lunch and a shift change of staff. The afternoon was siesta time, but still patients were brought in for admission and going to the operating theatre. There were relatives who kept vigil by the bedside of their loved ones. During the afternoon, I liked exploring the hospital corridors and gardens as I had so much time on my hands. I saw patients in a lot of pain. I saw young children with eye pads and some dragging their paralysed limbs.

I saw people sobbing and I heard the moaning of people who had lost their relatives. They had been to the *Mandir*, the Hindu temple, to pray and had a red mark with some rice on their forehead.

Outside, the gardens were dusty and the September dry weather left the ground parched and hard. Men sat in huddles smoking *bidis*, little rolled-up leaf cigarettes. I was fascinated with some men in the hospital garden who were smoking a *chillum*, a small hookah pipe. They would prod the embers until sparks flew about and the smoke swirled around them. The hospital garden had a peaceful corner with bougainvilia, jasmine and marigold, each of which had a strong fragrance. There were mango, tamarind and guava fruit trees. Parrots flew about pecking at the fruit. In the other corner of the lawn there were women making or preparing food for their relatives. These women had travelled to the hospital from their villages far away. Just outside the hospital gate there was a fruit and flower shop, where sometimes I could buy peanuts or peppermint sweets.

Often I would be sent by my fellow ward patients to bring boiled eggs, which the shop kept in a round wire container hanging outside. Flies buzzed all over the shop, in spite of the burning charcoal brazier, whose smoke was supposed to discourage them from coming near the food.

Evenings were full of relatives who brought food in tiffin-carriers: some brought fruit, some brought lemonade in bottles with a marble in the neck and some brought Vimto. Most evenings Bauji came to visit me, but occasionally he would send Brij. The food from home – *channa* and *puri*, stuffed vegetable paratha, – was delicious. Food provided by the hospital was basic but tasty. There was spiced lentil soup and mixed vegetable curry with rice. Very weak patients were given kedgeree – boiled rice and lentils mixed together with yogurt. My favourite food was double *roti*-toast, soaked in hot milk and sprinkled with sugar.

Night time had a life of its own. There were patients with oxygen cylinders making intermittent hissing and gurgling sounds. Some were in pain and were moaning and groaning. On occasion, everything usual would come to standstill when a seriously ill patient collapsed. Lights snapped on, trolleys were whisked up and down, and doctors rushed to revive the patient whilst nurses comforted relatives.

I became so friendly with staff that I helped roll washed cotton and crepe bandages for the ward. Sometimes they would tell me stories about Ali Baba and the Forty Thieves. Once in bed, I would put my plastered arm on a pillow beside me, covered in a rolled-up sheet. On many occasions I woke in the morning with a bruise on my face, having hit myself during the night.

I loved watching lizards running up and down the hospital walls, catching flies with one quick flick of their whip-like tongue. I watched spiders making their webs then awaiting their meal. After eight weeks I was discharged but went back for follow-up appointments. Three months after my surgery, the plaster was removed.

After my plaster was removed, The Prof came into the plaster room looking for me. "How is my junior assistant? You have been very brave. Now I can tell you will be able to do anything with your arm."

I was ecstatic and beaming with joy. I shook the Prof's hand saying "Thank you very, very much!" I had been practising saying this in English. Sister Margaret was with him and patted my head.

When Professor Roaf told me that the operation was a complete success and that my elbow's restricted movement would improve with time, I was overjoyed, and cried, and got a big hug from Sister Margaret. She said: *"Apne ko theek thak rakhna"* – "Keep you healthy." This was the last time I saw her, as she was returning to England with Professor Roaf. I have many happy memories of her, and thought at that time of the many kind and caring people in the world. Up until then, I had thought that you only get things done, or had people care for you, if you had money.

I was discharged from the hospital clinic to see my local bone specialist as necessary. I had to continue with my physiotherapy, and never saw Professor Roaf in India again. Over the years, every time I caught sight of my elbow, I remembered the great surgeon who saved me from such a hopeless situation. I told all my friends and relations about the Professor. He became my hero.

8: Lala Ka Baazar

WE HAD HAD ENOUGH mishaps in our haunted house, and Bauji made up his mind to move the family to a rented room in Lala Ka Bazaar, also in Meerut. We rented a room in a house near our uncle's house. Bauji was establishing a coal delivery business in partnership with Uncle, so the move made good sense. We rented a room on Nandi Street, the narrow passageway from Tehsil to Khanta Khar in the Lala Ka Bazaar area.

Telephone and electric cables criss-crossed the narrow alley like electrified wild spaghetti. The wires were just above our heads, within reach of an adult's raised hand. The tattered remains of dusty paper kites dangled from the network that stretched from wall to wall.

The houses were a mixture of red brick and stone. Most were single-storey and had flat concrete roofs, where the washing was hung out to dry. Our room was in a house made of brick; it had an entrance from a dark and narrow side street. The rickety wooden double doors led to a courtyard. Our room was off the courtyard. Beeji used a corner of our room, near the door, for the kitchen. She had very few utensils and did the cooking over a large bucket in which she had lit a coal fire. She cooked food sitting cross-legged on a low wooden stool. There were no chairs or table and we ate sitting on a *deri* spread out on the concrete floor. She cooked seasonal vegetables, lentils and rice. Sometimes we made coriander chutney, or we would have onion salad sprinkled with lemon juice and salt. At the other side of the courtyard, furthest away from our door, there grew a *neem* tree, one of the mahogany family, and beneath this, in the shade, was a hand pump. On the opposite side, a little concrete cubicle housed the latrine – a hole in the ground that we squatted over. A container beneath the hole was emptied daily by Sunder, the sweeper who lived nearby. He took the contents away in a basket lined with leaves that he hoisted onto his head. He left the latrine clean and smelling fresh with phenol.

We had four charpoy beds which had jute string stretched and interwoven into a pattern over a wooden frame, three feet wide by six feet long. I slept most of the time with my elder brothers, Raj or Brij, and my younger brother and sister slept together. In winter the charpoys were stacked up against the walls of the room, to give more space during the day. It was easy in the summer as all bedding was piled up outside in the courtyard. In the summer we slept in the courtyard or on the roof beneath the starry sky.

Our landlord and his wife were orthodox Hindu. Mrs Dutta wore her beautiful saris so that they covered her face all the time she was in public. We knew when she was coming, because her *panjam* ankle bracelet with small bells made a tinkling sound as she walked. Mr Dutta dressed in a *dhoti* loin cloth draped and folded to cover from his waist to below his knees. It was made from fine undyed homespun cotton, known as *khadi* cloth. A cotton thread hung from one shoulder to his opposite hip, to signify that he was of the Brahmin caste. His head was shaven except for a tuft of hair on the top of his head as a further sign of his learned Brahmin status.

The Lala Ka Bazaar was an area of dark, narrow streets, some of them only two to three metres wide, with three-storey buildings on each side. We boys would take a flying leap over the rooftops, from one side of the street to the other. I was always in trouble with my parents about this jumping. They were very protective of me because of my operation.

My friends Ramesh and Lovedev and I spent most of our time on the rooftops. Fearlessly flying from one building to another, we were the Kite Kings of our area. "Come on Ramesh, there's a big red one over there!" And we flew off in the direction of our prize, leaping from house top to house top, high above the street.

"Go on, Okhi, you can do it!" Lovedev would yell, as I teetered on the edge of a roof. I moved back a few paces and, crouching low, ran towards the gap. I took off with a flying leap and cleared the gap, landing on the roof next door.

"Go on, don't stop, get it, it's only over there!" So, on I ran, only stopping to take a few paces back, crouch low and gather speed for the next big leap. Ramesh and Lovedev were as keen as me and we would take a big jump with no thought of a fall or injury. To claim a kite whose string we had cut was the height of excitement for us, and we would seize our treasure from the roof before any of the other neighbourhood boys arrived to claim it.

One particular day, I took a flying leap without assessing the width of the gap. I missed my footing altogether, and caught the edge of the wall with my fingers. I clung on the wall for an eternity. I dangled above the electric wires and I pictured the street far below. I frantically grabbed the ledge with both hands. "Help!" I screamed. Fright gave me the strength to lever myself up and over the wall on to the flat rooftop. Unfortunately, I was seen and heard by someone who knew our family. My dangling act was described to my parents. "He's above Sudder Street, clinging on like a monkey two floors up!" When I got home, Father and Mother were waiting for me. I was given a shouting and I had to abandon this jumping adventure for a while.

There was open sewage on one side of the lane. The sewers were cleaned by sweepers and untouchables, but the place always stank, and we would hold our noses and walk quickly when passing by. Because the drains ran right alongside the house walls, no-one ever fell directly from the rooftop into the sewer. However, we did trip and fall in whilst playing in the road.

Ramesh, Lovedev and I had spotted a beautiful kite a few streets away. "Hey, Ram, let's get that beauty!" and with that the chase was on. We ran at breakneck speed down the street, ducking and diving between hawkers, rickshaws, debris and potholes. I ran looking skyward and did not see the cow in my path! With a slip of my sandals – which Father had made for all of us from old car tyres – and a twist of my ankle, I slipped over the slimy edge of the sewer and was knee-deep in thick stinking sewage. Momentarily I froze in horror. Ramesh and Lovedev had raced on and were nowhere in sight. I waded to the side through the rotting vegetables and foul water. I sat on the edge then swung my legs over the side and stood up. I stared at the blood running from cuts on my ankle and knee. I imagined the reception I would get from Mother and decided it was better not to go home until I had cleaned myself. I wandered around until I found a hand pump at the side of the street. I pumped hard and placed my legs under the running water. I stripped my tee-shirt off and soaked it as best as I could. My short trousers stank and I doused those while still wearing them. My sandals were good for any sort of rough treatment and underwent a good washing as well. As I wrung my thin cotton tee-shirt out and put it on my head to keep the sun off, I spotted Lovedev and Ramesh running up the street with the kite in their hands. The cuts were still oozing blood, so I gathered some dust from the road and put it on the cuts. I then spat on the palm of my hand and applied the saliva to the wounds. This treatment always seemed to work for our minor scrapes – I still have the scars to prove it.

"We'll stand in the sun a bit, so you can dry off, Okhi, and then we'll go home," Ramesh said, shaking the kite out. And that is what we did.

Some lanes had beautiful *haveli* houses, mansions with decorative entrances and beautiful murals of Hindu Gods or garden views. Sometimes on an outside wall there would be an alcove with a small Krishna statue covered with marigold flowers. There were large arched doors, often with brackets in the form of peacocks, decorating the hinges and handles. On Sundays these families would drive their horse-drawn carriages through the archways of their mansions and through the narrow lanes of our neighbourhood. We children were fascinated by the horses and the plumes of red or blue ostrich feathers on their heads. "Come on, Lovedev, let's follow them!" And we would march alongside the carriage wheels, scuffing up the dust as much as the horses' hooves.

Our house was not far from the area with rich merchants' mansions. There were two elephants near our street, used in transporting heavy weights such as bags of rice, wheat, cement or sugar cane. Our street elephants were docile, so we would feed them bananas, oranges or melons. They picked fruit very delicately from our hands and mostly we got a good lick as well.

There was always a large amount of elephant dung in the road. It had a strong smell, but not offensive. On unbearably hot days Ramesh would shout: "Hey, let's go to my house and pour water on the elephants!" We scampered up the stairs, collecting the Ramesh household buckets from their courtyard on the way. Leaning over the roof, we poured water on the elephants standing in the shade beneath. We knew the elephants loved our makeshift shower arrangements.

Ramesh, Lovedev and I helped Bablu and Rama, the *mahouts*, to wash their elephants in Surat Ganj. On the wide banks of Surat Ganj, we often saw gatherings of men who had come to pay their last respects to a departed relative. "Hari Krishna! Hari Rama! Hari, Hari Hari!" the relatives echoed the pundit, as the body, tightly wrapped in a white funeral cloth, was placed on the top of the funeral pyre. Surat Ganj Lake was where we all learned to swim.

The only time I have seen an elephant angry was when some stranger, for no good reason, hit him with a sharp piercing object. The elephant whipped around and, with ears held out and his head shaking from one side to the other, he thundered towards the person, chasing him into a doorway. The injured elephant lifted the door off its hinges and threw it on the courtyard cobbles. The door was smashed beyond repair. The mahout came running out and tenderly stroked his elephant's forehead and trunk. The mahout, in whom their elephants have supreme confidence, spent half an hour pacifying the animal.

One day an elephant lumbered through our narrow lane, carrying a load of bricks, completely blocking the way. So my friends and I crossed from one side of the lane to the other by passing between the elephant's legs. Elephants are revered by Hindus. They are the vehicle of Indra, the God of war, storms and rainfall. Sometimes they are painted and decorated with flowers and garlands to take part in religious processions. Decorated elephants are also sometimes used to carry the bridegroom to the bride's house on a wedding day.

In summertime the lanes got very dusty, so towards evening a man would walk the lanes, sprinkling water from a large sheepskin bag. I played in these lanes with my friends. Kanchan, an Indian version of marbles, was a favourite game, as it didn't need much space or money. Sometimes a well-off boy would bring a rubber ball and we would play with that, otherwise we would kick a tin can around, or play with whatever came to hand.

In the bazaar there was always something interesting. The narrow streets of Lala Ka Bazaar were full of potholes, traffic madness, sacred cows and hawkers. It ran from the closely packed Muslim area of Tehsil to the Khanta Khar, centre of Meerut city. It was a maze of lanes, so narrow that a cow and a person could hardly pass each other. There were braying donkeys carrying rice in jute bags; rickshaws piled high with schoolchildren; milkmen with 20-or-so milk churns clanking from the handlebars and any other accessible place on the bike; sleeping cows; a man carrying a big tin of ghee on his head; a woman in a long, swirling multi-coloured skirt balancing an enormous bundle of animal fodder on her head. Such was the traffic on Lala Ka Bazaar road.

Tiny wooden-fronted shops sold food, clothing, *masala* spice, *mathai* sweets. The masala shops had pyramids of red chillies, mounds of bright yellow turmeric, and heaps of black pepper corns, piled up on the counter. Jute bags of tamarind and dried coconut stood near the doorway. There were stacks of creamy-coloured cashew nuts, fragrant green cardamom pods, golden almonds and shrivelled dried dates.

In the jewellery quarter artisans sat cross-legged on small *deris* and moulded their precious and delicate wares over gas flames. Young lads fanned braziers of hot charcoal with bellows. Fumes, steam and dust covered the place. Sometimes the artisan was engulfed by clouds of steam, as he heated or cooled the gold. Close by were bigger workshops making, shaping and moulding brass trumpets, French horns and tubas. I loved sticking round to hear the musical notes being put to the test.

A small shop selling *paan* betel nut paste stood on the corner of the street and the alleyway, or *gali*. It could not have been more than one metre deep and two metres in length. The *paanwala* sat cross-legged on his cushion amongst his jars and leaves, a red spot on his forehead, as he had been to the temple. The aroma of betel nut, lime, cardamom, rose hip melba and chewing tobacco pervaded the air. There were snack vendors or *chaatwalas* every ten to fifteen metres, selling *samosas*, spiced potatoes, and *puris* sprinkled with chilli powder or tamarind sauce. Billboards on the shop walls reassured that real ghee was used in these premises. If a shopkeeper emptied dirty water on to the street, I would hop out the way.

The gun shops displayed double and single barrelled guns. A red cartridge belt was in the front of the largest shop window. Colourfully-clothed villagers smoked water-filled hookah pipes, which burned charcoal and tobacco. I loved passing the hookah shop as I watched the owner twirling and curling his very large moustache. Further down the street came the sweet shop where hot fresh *jelebi*, curled in a profusion of orange syrupy tubes on "plates" made from leaves. A huge black wok, one metre in diameter, sat over a fire and boiled milk until it thickened. The thickened milk *raberi*, sprinkled with split almonds, was served in conical brown clay pots. It was enticing to me but we could not afford these luxuries. Hawkers fanned the embers of their roadside braziers as they cooked sweet potatoes or *shakrkandi*, and sweet chestnuts or *singhara*.

A dental surgery displayed a poster which said *Teeth for life made here*. Two huge plastic dental plates hung outside and rattled in the wind. I was fascinated by a chap with long moustache and tight saffron coloured turban who cleaned customers' ears with probes, hooks and other gadgets which looked dangerous! On the days when the sweeper cleaned the drains, the road smelled of sewage. If we saw the sweeper cleaning the open drains, we would hold our nose and posh people put their handkerchiefs over their faces.

Because of the sugar cane growing in the fields around Meerut, the town was known for its freshly-made speciality sweets. Meerut's most famous confection is *raveri*, in which *gur* (raw sugar) is boiled to a semi-solid mass, and the whole elastic lump is either laboriously stretched between the arms of two sweet-makers or hung on two mechanical arms which rotate and stretch the hot gur until it resembles huge skeins of golden chewing gum. Small pieces are then hand-rolled and formed into tiny flat cakes and covered with sesame seeds. Another tasty sweet is *gajak*, which is unbelievably light and crumbly and tastes like a sort of golden ambrosia. Sweet shops also sold *barfi* and ruberi.

One of my favourite pastimes was watching monkeys as they jumped from house to house and down the lane. Often I would see a mother carrying her young baby, who clung to her chest or hung on her back near her head. The babies never lost their grip, and never had a fall. The monkeys called to each other in very high-pitched squeaky sounds, especially if there was danger around. They were quite adapted to their surroundings, living off food left out in the sunshine on the rooftops. They would even dare to go into the compound and steal food from the larder or kitchen, or fruit from a table inside the rooms. I often pulled silly faces at them and they would copy it back to me. I tried to catch a baby monkey, but without success. I used to annoy the monkeys by reflecting the sun into their eyes with a mirror. Sometimes they would throw a stone at me. They were fond of clothes, and would often pull them from the washing line and try on a shirt or a petticoat. If you wanted the garment returned, the trick was to put on a similar garment, then slowly remove it and throw it on the ground. The monkey would then do the same, and then you had to be quick to retrieve the article.

Our next-door neighbours, Naresh and Seema Sharma, were a young couple who had married two years previously and were blessed with a beautiful son. Naresh had a jewellery shop in the bazaar. Beeji, as an experienced mother, often went to help Seema with her new baby. Seema was very shy and wore her sari covering her head and partly her face. But I had seen her long dark hair flowing in the air.

One day, up on the flat roof, the child lay on a charpoy, flinging his legs in the air and making gurgling noises whilst Seema nearby hung washing to dry on the metal line. Monkeys, as usual, were all around. A neighbour on the opposite side was feeding fruits to the monkeys.

Without warning, a monkey snatched the new baby from his cot and scampered over to the edge of the roof overlooking the street. The monkey kept a close grip on the baby, and by now everyone, including the baby, was screaming. Seema screamed at the top of her voice and shouted: "Monkey has taken my baby! He will kill him! For God's sake do something!" With tears all over her face, she screamed towards Mother for help: "Please get Naresh from the shop!" Everybody came up on their roof to see the commotion and started yelling at the monkey without much avail. Beeji sent Brij to the bazaar to fetch Naresh.

All the neighbours were on their roof to give any help they could. Mrs Gupta, living on the other side of our house, a widow dressed in a white sari and with silver hair, brought a doll onto the roof. First, she made little rocking movements and then placed the doll very gently on the floor. To everyone's astonishment, the monkey also made little rocking movements whilst cradling the baby, and then it laid the infant very tenderly on the rooftop and walked away. Cries of happiness and gasps of relief went round the assembled crowd and our neighbours thanked God and Mrs Gupta for such a happy ending to the incident. There was great rejoicing in the street and Seema and Naresh gave everyone sweets.

At the far end of Lala Ka Bazaar's narrow lanes was the Tehsil area of Meerut city. It was the Muslim area. Tehsil was darker, narrower and more densely packed than our area of town. It was also filthy.

This was the time when the Partition of India had only recently taken place. There were old scores to be settled between Hindus and Muslims. One afternoon I was playing with my friend near our house when a crowd of Sikhs, brandishing swords, came down the street towards us. They yelled at us to go into a house, shut the door and not to come out again. There was a procession of fifteen Sikhs with long beards, dressed in navy *kurta* pajamas with navy turbans. The shiny swords in their hands flashed in the shafts of light. They had saffron scarves round their necks and all were chanting loudly: "*Wah Guru, wah Guru!*" – Praise to the Guru, their religious leader. I could recognise some of them as our neighbours.

Hindus joined them and had daggers in their hands, hiding them behind their backs so we children would not see. They were shouting: "Kali, Hindu Goddess of fierce warriors, will kill these bastards!" They all looked fierce with their weapons and some had latti bamboo sticks ready to beat someone. They were shouting: "Revenge! These bastards have to be given a lesson!"

We ran to my house and told Bauji and Beeji what we had seen and that the Sikhs had said we were not to come out on the street again that day. We were scared. Bauji and Beeji said there was going to be trouble. "Nobody is going out! Rival gangs will be roaming the streets and looking for revenge!" Father shouted across the room.

School was cancelled and we were banned from going on the roof of the house as Bauji knew a killing was likely. The following day we heard a man had been killed in a lane outside our house. Bauji told us that Muslims had abducted a Hindu man from Tehsil district and decapitated him on the street and set fire to his body. Killing a Muslim was the revenge. Afterwards there was a dried blood stain on the large stone covering the drains and I saw large red blobs in the drains near the stone and bloody markings on the stone across the street, as if a body had been dragged across. The person killed was a Muslim shopkeeper known to Bauji in the vegetable market.

There were riots all over Meerut with looting and burning of houses and shops. This lasted for five days. We were surrounded by police. A police officer in a rickshaw urged people to be calm and peaceful and said police were there to help everybody.

We as a family had gone through hell and were very anxious, living close to a Muslim district. We even thought of going back to Delhi to be in a secure place. We did not go to school for a long time and I did not venture to play outside on the street for months.

More problems were on the way. When Kuckoo was five years old, he suddenly developed a fever. His temperature was 105 Fahrenheit and my parents thought we might lose him. Two days before, we had been to the market and had had a rare treat of large crisps, puffed up and filled with spicy water – *pani puri*. Kuckoo became delirious and was so ill that he could not lift his head from the pillow. He had a tummy ache and rashes on his chest. He passed rice-water stools, which looked like dishwater. He coughed persistently and kept us all awake. He looked yellow, his eyes sank into the back of his head and his lovely curly hair was plastered with sweat. We took turns in fanning him with a hand-held fan, and we sponged him with pieces of ice, cut from a big block by the ice vendor in the street.

Dr Chopra came to see Kuckoo at home and diagnosed typhoid fever. We could not afford to take him to a private hospital, so Mr Shivastava, the chemist, made up doses of chloramphenicol. Mr Shivastava came twice daily to give Kuckoo the antibiotic by injection. Beeji went into action, overseeing hygiene of food, water and hand washing. All our drinking and cooking water was thoroughly boiled. Water used for washing spoons and plates and clothes was chlorinated first. The room was washed with phenol two or three times every day and the drains were washed thoroughly and treated with DDT. Beeji paid the sweeper a little extra cash to keep the outside drains clean. She was awake all hours of the day and night.

Kuckoo was still going downhill fast. I told Ramesh and Lovedev: "He is getting more delirious and his temperature will not come down, even though we put ice-cold sponges on his forehead." He developed blood in his motions. We prayed every day and asked our priest to pray with us in the house. We dared not eat without washing our hands until they were nearly washed away. We were barred from eating anything but home-cooked food. Mother cooked lentils, rice and non-spicy vegetables.

Kuckoo's temperature gradually began to settle down and he became a bit more alert. He was very thin and weak, but gradually he began to take an interest in life again. I started playing card games with him. After about six weeks, we knew that Kuckoo would survive. To thank God for his blessing, we arranged a thanksgiving ceremony, burning wood sticks with clarified butter and incense, a *havan* in the Arya Samaj. After the ceremony, we distributed God-blessed food, *prasad*, to the entire congregation and to our friends and neighbours.

9: Food and Drink

WE OFTEN STROLLED into town and down the High Street after our evening meal, meeting with other families, also strolling in the cool of the evening. The groups we met would often number eight or ten from four generations of one family. Shops and markets were open as late as the demand lasted, usually until around eleven at night, and in my childhood they were softly lit by the kerosene lamps hung from low ceilings. They made an interesting hissing noise and had a warm smell.

Making for the *paan* stall was an after-dinner ritual. Paan is a blend of menthol, lime, betel nuts, sugar, sweet melba and maybe ginger and cardamom. The exact proportions are to the paan maker's own recipe, and everyone has their own favourite paan maker. Ours would park his handcart in his usual place and sit in the yellow glow of two paraffin lamps suspended above the cart. He sat cross-legged in the middle of the cart, his jars of ingredients stacked up behind him, his bare feet in the paan leaves. The leaves were soaked in a basin of water, shaken dry and held in his cupped hand. He then selected from his jars the ingredients for either sweet paan, ordinary paan or paan with tobacco, according to the customer's request. A teaspoonful of the concoction was placed on the leaf which was then folded to make a bite-sized parcel and finally wrapped in newspaper.

One of the ingredients of paan stains bright red everything with which it comes into contact, and – since the correct way to eat paan is to pop it into your mouth in one go and hold it in the inside cheek for leisurely chewing – it has plenty of time to stain teeth, tongue and lips a florid red, so we always made a point of smiling broadly at everyone we met as we wandered home. And after the chewing, came the spitting. Everywhere we made bright red spit marks – along the streets, up on the walls and on doorsteps. I have never seen ladies spit – they must swallow – but we males spat very noisily.

I was also very fond, especially in the summer months, of *shikangvi,* a drink made from freshly-squeezed lemon and crushed ice, together with water and sugar. Sometimes, to enhance the taste, we would add some salt and pepper. Shikangvi is usually served at teatime in very hot weather and is very refreshing. I never got enough of it – with my brothers and sisters all wanting it too, we didn't get huge amounts, and it was all the more tasty because we as a family did not have it very often. It was normally served to guests, as we didn't have bottled drinks.

Another drink, *ruafsa*, is one that we only had in the house when relatives or guests were visiting. Red in colour, it is made of *khus khus* and other aromatic ingredients, mixed with corn sugar syrup and diluted with water. It is considered to be a good, cooling drink on a hot day but I had it only once, on an occasion when we had guests

I was intrigued by the spiced water vendor, whom I saw throughout my young life. He was a small, very thin old gentleman dressed in khadi clothes comprising kurta and dhoti, the traditional Hindu dress for men. He was kind and gentle. He carried a clay pot in a jute sack slung under his left arm, and served spicy water in containers made from the peepul tree leaves, which he had pinned together with wooden twigs. He would often add some spicy chutney made from coriander, green chillis, *imli* (tamarind) juice, salt and other spices. We would drink and enjoy it by blowing out our breath to get rid of the heat of the chillis. It would cost us only a few *annas*, the lowest denomination in Indian currency.

Hot roasted peanuts were a treat in the winter months. The vendor roasted them over charcoal in a clay pot and carried them in a jute sack under his armpit. I never worked out how he never got burned. The vendor sold the peanuts in their shells, and they were delicious, particularly on a winter evening or late at night. The vendor had his special way of letting us know that he was around: he shouted *Mungphaliwala!* on the street corner. His was the cheapest snack, and we could usually afford it.

Ice cream was not readily available, because it was too expensive, but ice lollies were. On very hot days we would find a vendor sitting on a wooden cart under the shade of a tree, with large pieces of ice covered in jute sacking, so that they would not melt. He would make crushed ice by shaving the ice with a wood-plane. A large peepul tree leaf was placed underneath, to catch the shavings. He would ask which colour syrup we would like. I often had red, blue *and* green.

Chaat is a very hot and spicy delicacy which I was not interested in as a child. But later I acquired the taste and could not get enough of it.

Golguppa is large bubbles of crispy deep-fried batter, and its hollow centre is filled with spiced water. It was my favourite snack: I could eat six at a time and would have liked more, and it was a great feeling to be blowing out my hot breath because of the chilli effect.

Occasionally we would buy *tikki* (round mashed potato with a spicy part in the middle) which I liked roasted on the *tava* (iron griddle) and sprinkled with yogurt, imli, chutney and crushed or dried chilli.

We would always have proper *chai* at our house. It is made with proper tea leaves, full cream milk, water and spices including *elichi* (cardamom) *somf* (aniseed) and *long* (cloves), all boiled and strained. Sometimes we would ask for ten-mile tea, so-called because it could keep you refreshed, full and satisfied while walking on your journey for the next ten miles. It is traditionally served in little throwaway clay pots, but nowadays small glasses set on a saucer have replaced them. I always poured my tea into the saucer to cool it down as I was not good at drinking tea, which would scald my fingers and tongue. In the evening I would call on my friend Kamlesh with a "Go for a chai at Begum Bridge?" We would call for other friends, like Rajesh and Davinder, and the four of us would sit there discussing politics, gossip, read newspapers and exchange notes about girls. There was always the sound of *"Chai! Garam Chai!"* ("Tea! Hot tea!") all around, as the chaiwalas brought the trays of chai.

Another food I enjoyed was sugar cane. Meerut is the heart of the sugar cane growing area, so it was easily available in the season. I would go with my friends to Begum Bridge where cartloads of sugar cane were on their way to the sugar factory. Sneaking up behind the cart and pulling a few canes out of the load, we could peel the cane with our teeth and chew and suck the juice. It was sweet and fresh; and, being stolen goods, cost nothing and was even sweeter.

In the winter months there was roasted corn on the cob, cooked over charcoal and made tastier by dipping it in lime juice, then sprinkling salt and chilli powder. I enjoyed watching it being roasted over the sparkling charcoal with the crackling noises. It gave me a warm sensation and made me feel hungry. I can remember one occasion when, being very greedy and having had four roasted cobs which I had stolen from the field, I ended up with a real tummy ache!

In summer it was a delight to see huge green water melons, cut in half and displayed along the road. We had water melon in season and ate it after lunch at high noon. We children looked forward to it and finished our food quickly to get the juicy bright red pieces. We devised a trick to get melon which was being transported on a cart. We would deliberately walk in front of the bullock, causing the driver to pull up sharp in the middle of the road, dislodging two or three water melons, which then fell on the road and split open. The *cartwala* would not bother to gather them up again and we would eat our split water melon under the trees in the park.

In early summer, mangoes were at a premium and very expensive. I didn't venture as far as buying them. We would often secretly climb a tree in the nearby orchard and pick unripe mangoes which were green and not really edible, but I was very fond of the sharp taste when it was eaten with salt and masala. As the season progressed, however, mangoes became less expensive, so Bauji would bring some home most lunch times and we would eat them with our meal. It was a great feast. I became very good at eating the stone of the mango fruit, as I could have as many stones as I liked. On our picnics we would put mango and water melon in a jute bag and tie the bag to a stone in the river; and then, when we were hungry a few hours later, enjoy eating the cold fruits.

At the end of the summer, we started seeing the small *desi* mango, which cannot be cut. The best time to buy quantities of the small mango was at the start of the monsoon season; we would eat them in the street, walking in the rain and enjoying our treat as we got splashed in the puddles. Eating mango in the monsoon rain was actually encouraged, to get rid of the prickly heat and spots caused by the hot summer. In late summer there were also small green and yellow mangoes called *chusa,* the size of a large hen's egg. We would hold one in the palm of our hand and squeeze on all sides, then bite the top off the mango where it had been attached to the tree, and suck out all the juice. Once finished, we would suck on the stone to get every bit of the flesh. We would even roast the stone and break it open to get the fleshy seed, which was bitter – but when put with drinking water, it tasted sweet and delicious.

So many simple pleasures, which cost us very little!

10: Local Amusements

IN EARLY CHILDHOOD I was immersed in playing games
with my friends and keeping myself busy outside the house,
investigating anything and everything. To amuse myself, I had a
metal bicycle wheel frame without any spokes, which I moved
along with a round piece of wood, running along beside it as fast
as I could. My friends and I thought it was brilliant.

Night-time was magical, especially in the summer when
there was a full moon. After our meal outside in the courtyard,
we would be out on the street to play hide and seek, or we visited
neighbours to catch up with news. We loved to be under the trees
as the cold bright moonlight flickered and sprinkled patterns
over our faces. Sometimes we could hear birds rustling in the
branches overhead. We would chase each other around the
courtyard, in and out of the shadows. The moon occasionally slid
behind the clouds, reappearing minutes later. It was fantastic. My
favourite trip was to the paan shop on Gurdwara Road, a popular
place for lots of families to meet regularly and pass on messages.
Back home later, tired out and ready for bed, it was wonderful to
settle in the moonlight and be together with the family, chatting
about interesting things that had happened in school and amongst
our friends.

Our older brothers would tell us younger ones stories of
Ali Baba and the Forty Thieves, or about movies they had seen,
or even make up their own tales. Our imaginations would run
wild as we thought of exciting adventures, and in turn we would
tell stories of the jungle, lions, leopards, elephants and talking
birds. One particular story revolved around a baby girl lost in the
jungle and taken away by a monkey. The parents were unable to
find their baby, but all the while she was being looked after in
the jungle by the monkey, which took care of her as if she were
its own. The child started living like an animal and developed a
bushy head and lots of body hair and could climb like an animal.
One day some humans saw the child, but no-one could catch her.
This turned out to be based on a true story of an incident near
Lucknow. We heard that the little girl was eventually rescued
from the jungle but had significant problems in adjusting to life
as a human being, unable even to sleep on a charpoy or sit on a

chair. She would rather sit and sleep on the floor, and ate like an animal. I don't remember what happened after that, but I do remember sometimes, before drifting into sleep, I thought that I could have been in the jungle with that little girl.

The next thing we knew it would be early morning with the sun shining down on us. We would get up and clear away our bedding and put the charpoy on its side against the wall near the house.

In summer the heat was intense, and most people would only go out for a few minutes, but that was not for me. I was still going about all my activities, kite flying and playing games, under the glare of the noonday sun. Beeji was always warning us that we would get sunstroke, and on occasion we would heed her advice, but often the temptation was just too much. I remember a friend who basked in the sun and developed sunstroke. He was taken to hospital for a week and put on a drip, losing a lot of weight as he could not eat or drink.

The *loo* is a feature of the hot midsummer. It is a very hot and dusty wind like the fiery blast from an oven, fiercely blowing into every corner and crevice, and there is no escape from it. If we did go outside, we had to put a handkerchief over our nose and mouth, and cover our eyes with our hands. It really was very troublesome, as some loo periods could last three or four weeks and prevent us from playing out.

We were very aware of the films in cinema halls in the town. Seeing a Bollywood movie is an experience that takes the whole evening. First comes the getting ready and the dressing up in best clothes, the film, the interval, the pre-, post- and half-way through snacks. Bollywood films always last about three hours. The whole family goes, with infants and children slung over the parents' shoulders. The story line always follows a familiar pattern, incorporating religious and romantic aspects, and always, at the end, culminating in good triumphing over evil. The shows were full of songs, were overacted and had predictable jokes from the same well-known actors. There was a lot of yelling, crying, punching and impossible hardships in the film, but it always came out right in the end. There was much getting-up and going-out and coming back with food throughout the film and a good deal of munching and unwrapping of paper during the show.

Intermissions were always long and we would all go out to the vendors waiting outside in the street with hot roasted chick peas and fried potato tikki pasties. Some vendors had a brazier with a cast iron griddle making spicy tamarind-flavoured chaat. There would be a row of men lined up near a drain pipe outside the cinema hall relieving themselves. Loudspeakers carried crackling film music. Huge posters of leading actors were posted all over the walls outside, sometimes even incorporating flashing lights.

11: A Camel Never Forgets

FATHER HAD A COAL BUSINESS. He took delivery of coal at the railway siding. I was recovering from my arm operation and Bauji used to take me with him so that I would not get bored at home or think too much about my arm. Bauji's business was in an industrial area where every kind of transport was coming and going. Trucks, horns blaring, belched fumes. Bullock-carts, camel-carts and donkeys all seemed to be engaged in an eternal journey. There were shoals of cyclists, deaf dogs, sudden crossing of goats, all jockeying for position. Tractors pulled carts of hay as large as a moving hillside.

I was fascinated by the camels. Their height and hump and their delicate way of stooping down to offload the delivery delighted me. They were always doing a chewing action with a side-to-side movement of the jaw, and there was always lots of froth coming from the mouth. The camels were controlled by a ring through the nose with a rope on their mane. The *camelwalas* were very gentle people and treated their camels well. I used to love seeing the camels being ridden. On winter evenings, as the sun went down, a haze of smoke from the fires cooking evening meals rose and added to the clouds of dust kicked up by the camel herds returning home. The air would be so thick that only their silhouettes were visible.

In Lala Ka Bazaar there was a herd of 30 camels, their spindly legs strode in unison. They transported bags of wheat and rice to markets in the city. Father employed two brothers, Badlu and Kalu, in his coal business. I often spent time with them and they knew Mohan the camelwala well. "Can I ride a camel and feed them?" I asked Badlu. He took me over to where the camels rested.

Mohan, dressed in a dusty cotton shirt and pyjama trousers, sandals made from old car tyres on his feet, threw a green shawl around his head and face and rose from his haunches, shook the reins and said: "Cluck, cluck, cluck!" The camel folded his legs and I was lifted on his back. I clung to the hump while the camel heaved himself up. He began a slow and bumpy walk, but quickly gathered pace, and soon we were kicking dust in great clouds behind us as we sped along at breakneck speed. I was exhilarated, with my shirt flying behind me and the dust making my hair stand on end and my eyes water. I felt breathless, as if everything was shaken up inside me.

Finally my camel came to a sudden halt and decided to nibble the thorny leaves of an acacia tree growing nearby. He lifted his head so suddenly that he jerked me backwards, so I had to hold on to the rein. Kalu gave me an armful of fodder from a huge pile of greens he had chopped with his hand-driven machine.

"Have you ever been kissed by a camel?" Mohan asked as he arranged the rein and, petting the camel on his nape, he whispered something to the camel. The animal leaned towards me and gave me a kiss on my cheek, leaving a large slick of saliva all over the side of my face. When the camel had settled comfortably, sitting with its legs folded underneath, Mohan squatted beside the camel with a twinkle in his eye and reached underneath it. "Open your mouth, Okhi!" and he squirted milk into my mouth from the udders. The milk was warm, slightly salty and tasty.

All the herders were squatted down beside a fire they had lit to cook their evening meal. The elder herders chatted whilst the young apprentices saw to the camel fodder and water. A hookah pipe, smoking and gurgling as it was passed around the circle, added to the smoke that swirled all over. As dusk descended and the air grew cooler, the herders huddled closer to the fire. Time passed quickly and it would soon be time for Bauji to finish work and then we would be heading for home.

On one occasion we witnessed the unthinkable – a camelwala beating and violently pulling the ring of his camel. Bauji was incensed and shouted: "Hey you! What do you think you are doing to that poor camel?"

Father often told me that a camel has a very long memory and that they do not forget anything done to them. I did not believe this and always thought the camel to be a docile animal. A few months later, however, we were in Bauji's business area and suddenly there was a great deal of commotion and people were screaming. We ran towards the crowd and saw a camel had hold of a man's neck in his jaw. The camel would not let go and nobody could stop the animal, even though everybody was hitting it with bamboo sticks. The camel only released the man's neck after the victim had died of suffocation. The crowd were discussing how the camelwala had been cruel so many years before. They were saying: "The camel has a long memory; you will pay the price for any misdeeds sooner or later."

This was the very same camelwala to whom Bauji had shouted for hitting the camel!

12: A Man Called Mamaji

WE CALLED MOTHER'S BROTHER MAMAJI. Uncle's real name was Dharam Pal, although he liked to be called Mr Pal. From as far back in my childhood as I remember, he was a domineering man. It was he who advised our family to settle near him in Meerut. Mother wanted to be near some relatives after the partition of India, and so we came to live in Meerut.

Mamaji was a round-bellied man. He had a plump face, small teeth, owlish eyes framed by his round spectacles. He was always dressed in western-style clothes, a suit and tie topped off with a Kashmiri fur cap, in winter and summer. He was a loud, boastful man, full of himself. He talked constantly about the *shikars* (hunts) with his friends. He boasted to all in the family about how much money he had made. At one time we hired a one-bedroom place near to Mr Pal. It was in the compound near the Lala Ka Bazaar area in Meerut City. We were one of four families in the house, living under one communal roof.

Mamaji had set up a coal business with my Bauji. We all thought Mr Pal was very helpful at first. But gradually we noticed that he did not put any work into the business and eventually did not even turn up for work. Bauji did everything, but Mamaji still demanded half the profits. As children, we did not realise what was happening, but as we became older we persuaded Bauji to raise this with Mamaji.

We wanted Bauji to stop paying him any money from the coal business. But Bauji, being Bauji, evaded the issue and carried on as usual; he didn't want the fight or the hassle, and Mamaji knew this and took full advantage of it. It took me and my brothers many years to persuade Bauji to stop the payments and I am still not sure that they stopped completely. I felt so strongly about it that I asked Beeji to confront her brother, and over time we stopped socialising with him and his family.

Mamaji was always making waves and arguments within the family. He would say: "How's my *bachen* (child)?"

"I am doing fine," I would reply to Mamaji.

"You should come and work with me, college is no good, it's a waste of time!"

"You are talking nonsense, education is very important!" Beeji would retort angrily.

"Look, I've always been your well-wisher; you can't talk to me like that!" Mamaji would say, and then go into a huff and he would get up and leave our house.

"He is well known within our family for being a man whose mouth is two steps ahead of his head," Beeji would say.

We discovered that, when we all had to flee over the border, Mamaji's elder sister, our auntie, had given him money to buy a house for her and her husband in Meerut, near to Mamaji. He bought the council house with her money and lived in it himself! She put her life savings into the purchase, and he claimed the house in his own name. My aunt and uncle, whom I had visited in Sardhana, were left homeless by his actions and we children could not understand how a brother could behave like this towards his sister.

I never forgave him. And from my college days onwards, I never visited him again.

13: Flying Kites

I HAD BECOME a *patang baaz* – a kite fanatic.

Kite-flying, my favourite hobby, was to bring me a championship.

My interest started when we were living at Lala Ka Bazaar where, because the lanes were very narrow – about two to three metres wide – we spent most of our time on the roof. I was particularly fascinated by big colourful kites high up in the sky.

I would fly my own small kite with my right hand, as my left arm was in plaster, and everyone was amazed by my skill in one-handed kite-flying. I was often in trouble with Beeji and Bauji for climbing on our roof and jumping from one roof to another, with no thought of safety, in the hope of finding a cut kite and getting it for nothing. I loved the tilting of the kite from side to side and particularly the paper-bird-flapping-its-wings sound. Later, I became a champion kite flyer and could compete with the best. I was seen everywhere flying kites.

Naturally, after a while I wanted to be able to make my own kites. I went to the *kitewala* to see how they were made. I started making my own with newspapers and twigs from Beeji's sweeping broom. I learned how to balance the kite and how to manoeuvre it. I made my own glue, mixing together a paste of self-raising flour or tree resin and water. It would keep for a few days in a small cup sealed with paper. I used old newspapers to make my kites, strengthening and reinforcing them with extra snippets of newspaper. I would have preferred tissue paper, but it was difficult to get and was expensive.

After the construction of the kite came the balancing. Out to an open space I would go, and by lengthening or shortening the top and bottom cotton threads to get the balance just right, my kite became very manoeuvrable. I was then ready for the trial run.

With the spool in my hand, I ran into the wind. I could feel the kite lift and tug at the string. I played out more string from the spool as my newspaper kite soared up, up and away into the wide blue yonder. My tactic of tugging sharply on the string, using strong quick arm movements, lifted the kite high above the rooftops, catching the hot dry thermals as they swirled around above the plains. Once up there, my kite would stay steadily on the thermals for hours, making wonderful flapping noises, which was music to my ears.

As I became more successful, I began to put my kite up to join the flying battles that raged on the rooftops nearly every day. Many kites would be fluttering aloft, but this was no pretty spectacle, this was war. The idea was to cut your opponent's kite string with *your* string. In order to do that, the string had to be coated in glass-powder. To begin with, I could not afford the powdered glass-covered thread, so I developed a way of making my own. I would smash a glass bottle, and my sister and I would pound the pieces of glass to a fine dust. We would coat sewing cotton thread with a mixture of glass powder and my own flour and glue mixture – and many times we cut ourselves making glass-covered thread, which is officially known as *manjha*.

Manjha is used to cut other kites by several techniques. Sometimes the weight of the kite could be harnessed, or it could be done by the sudden change in angle of the kite. I spent long hours watching these manoeuvres in great excitement and anticipation. Cutting a kite was exciting, and I was always running around to claim these cut kites, my family and friends watching in horror as I leapt three or four feet at a time from one rooftop to another high above the street. Obviously I was in constant trouble with my parents, especially as my arm was still in plaster. Sometimes when flying my kite, I would try to anchor the cut kite by intricate movements of my own kite around the thread of the cut one. Once both were anchored, I could bring them both down. When sand storms or dust storms blew, I would get my kite into the eye of the whirlwind and it would soar higher and higher without effort, and I would imagine how wonderful it would be if only I could go up into the clouds with it.

I looked forward to the Basant festival. On this day families celebrate and rejoice the start of spring and local kite-flying competitions are held. The sky is speckled with kites of every size and colour. I had been preparing my kites and manjha as soon as I returned home from school. It had become my ritual. There was fierce competition from Audu, Ramesh Bishnoi and a well-known kite guru from the market called Babu. One year I had beaten Babu and the next year he was out to reclaim his title as undisputed kite champion.

Basant day arrived and the sky was a cloudless bright blue. A light breeze blew, perfect for kite flying. My friends and I were dressed in our brightest clothes and I had slicked my hair down with Bauji's Brylcreem. Kuckoo, my staunch supporter, was with me on the rough, barren, potholed land at the back of our house.

"Come on, let's start the kite flying and show them what we're made of!" my little brother yelled. Kuckoo ran on ahead and lifted the kite on his head ready for launching. He put his finger in the air and tested the breeze and then gave a pull on the manjha twice to let me know he was ready. He shouted: "Breeze from over your right shoulder! Are you ready?"

I was looking up to the sky to see if any other kite was going to obstruct mine. I gave a good tug and I felt the gust of wind take my kite shimmering up into the sky, making a mighty roaring noise as it sailed higher and higher. Kuckoo returned and patted my back, saying "We will beat the lot today!"

Shashi jumped up and down and tugged on my sleeves, wanting to hold the kite. "I want to fly the kite and sweep it down on Sushma's house!" The wind was getting stronger, perfect for cutting kites, and I was able to get my kite high in the sky. I gave the kite spool to Shashi and she screamed with excitement as she was pulled forward by the strength of it. Audu had already launched his trademark green kite from his rooftop, which gave him an advantage of panoramic views of the whole sky, sweeping low down over trees. He was lifting, diving and looping with great skill. Kuckoo told me that he had already cut ten kites.

Suddenly a huge red-and-white-striped kite swept overhead, threatening our territory. I kept a close eye on him. This was Babu from the market showing me that he was ready to compete. I noticed lots of my friends and other boys and girls looking toward the sky. I knew the fight was on. "Give me more manjha, Kuckoo! I must get higher!" I roared.

Out of the corner of my eye, I saw Ramesh running very fast after a spinning kite on the street. "You must keep your eyes on the sky!" Kuckoo shouted. In that split second, I cut my finger as the manjha unwound under tension on the reel. Big red drops of blood flowed onto the spool and landed in the dust on the ground near my feet. I sucked my finger; there was no time to worry about that.

"Okhi! Look out! Look out! Babu is coming towards you!" Kuckoo and Shashi screamed together. I was ready for it, as I turned my kite toward Babu's to test his move. He dived low over the trees and high buildings, sweeping under my kite at an acute angle. I lowered my kite with full tension. He realised that his move was not going to be successful and he retreated to his territory. For a long time there was a cat-and-mouse game but, with the help of a strong wind and a straight lift, I finally managed to nail his kite. Fatally injured and rudderless, it floated like a dead bird, flopping one side, then the other, to the ground. Children on the street scampered to claim the orphan kite.

My friends on the rooftops, heads poking through windows and above high parapets, shouted: "Hurray! You did it, Okhi!"

Kuckoo and Shashi jumped up and down, throwing fists in the air, screaming "You are the kite guru! You have proved it, Patang Baaz!"

I felt great. A fast thumping sensation began in my chest. Brij, who had been witnessing the kite fight from the rooftop, turned up on my patch and thumped me on my back. "Well done!" he grinned.

Kuckoo, running towards the enormous red and white striped kite as it spiralled down, disappeared from my side for half an hour or more. When he returned, he presented me with my trophy, Babu's kite.

I started bringing my own kite down, Shashi turning the spool, until all my precious manjha had been wound back. I swaggered down the street as if I had won an Olympic medal, with a huge grin on my face and my bony little chest stuck out a mile. Kuckoo, my biggest fan at that moment, trotted along beside me telling everyone we met that I had won the tournament.

I loved flying my kite at night to show off my kite control to friends and competitors. There were younger kids in our courtyard who were thrilled to hold the kite late in the evening with darkness closing in. I would tie the string to the leg of a charpoy and let it fly for hours in the night. It was a great feeling to put the kite in front of a full moon and make a print on the moon and a shadow on the ground. On occasion, I would fly the kite the whole night without touching it. I started sending some balloons high in the sky attached to the string, which was amusing to my brothers and sister. I decided to send lanterns lit with *devas*, small oil-filled clay pots with a wick. It was thrilling to see a lighted lantern dangling in the dark sky without any support. But one night the lantern caught fire and the string was cut. I lost the kite and the devas dropped from the sky on a lady neighbour's head and her clothes were aflame. Luckily it was put out by Beeji and Shashi smothering the clothes. But then I was in real trouble and I was banned from night kite flying.

14: Holiday in Sardhana

WE DID NOT HAVE MANY HOLIDAYS – we could not afford them. But one summer my Beeji thought it would be a good idea for me to spend some time with Jagat Priya Mehta, my uncle. He lived in Sardhana, some 20 miles from Meerut. My aunt Indravati was my mother's eldest sister, my *masiji* or maternal aunt. She had taken my mother under her wing years ago when they lost their Beeji. My mother had been only three years old when she lost *her* mother and Indravati looked after her.

My parents had written a letter to my uncle two months earlier to ask if I could visit them for two weeks in the summer. Brij put me on a bus, and my uncle picked me up at the other end of my journey. "Beta ka kia hal hai!" Uncle said as I stepped down from the bus, "How are you, son?" And he took my very small attaché case, the only case my family owned. "We are looking forward to having you, you'll enjoy village life," he said, as he gave me a big squeeze. The road was on high ground banked up on both sides. We descended steeply downhill to Uncle Jagat's house.

The village was made of baked mud. Small single-storey houses, walls around the courtyards, the well in the centre of the village, even the square in the centre of the village, were all made from the same beige-coloured mud. Imprints of the hands in the wet mud that formed the walls made pleasing patterns. All the constructions had soft fluid lines, corners were rounded so no wall was straight or angular. Men on bicycles wobbled along the main street, ringing their bells. Women carried huge bundles of sugarcane leaves on their heads. I saw conical shaped towers covered with reeds dotted around the village. There were stacks of cow dung, patted into flat pancakes and stacked away for fuel, as wood piles are stacked in the west. There was a goat herder looking after his flock. The goats were very agile, jumping and flinging their hind legs. A dozen curious children walked in front of us, eager to talk to me. We were stopped a number of times to exchange greetings.

"This is my pharmacy," Uncle Jagat pointed to a small room on the main road. "*Namaste,* Doctorji!" the shopkeepers said. The meaning of "Namaste" is "I will take your dust on to me" and it is a polite *hello* in Hinduism. We wandered through the narrow lane of the village until we came to uncle's house. It was late in the afternoon and villagers were returning to work after siesta. It was still very hot and Uncle had a black umbrella to protect us from the sun. I already had sweat patches under my arms.

Uncle Jagat was a very learned man; he had a degree in Sanskrit as well as a great command of Hindi. He was a scholar in Ayurvedic medicine and had set up a dispensing practice in the village. He wore *kurta* pyjamas of homespun cloth and had a cap of the same fabric.

I was recovering then from the surgery on my broken elbow and uncle was very gentle, dressing my arm in khaki cloth. I had become interested in medicine because of my broken arm and what I had seen and experienced during my long hospital stay. My uncle showed me all his potions, ointments and herbal medicinal treatments, and allowed me to sit with him while he was consulting or dispensing. He showed me the herbs he used in different ointments and how he used to make mixtures of leaves, roots and gur for treating patients with chest problems. I remember one particular very effective remedy which was used universally for headache, tummy ache, diarrhea, toothache and joint pain, as well as an antiseptic. This was *amrithara*, which he made from camphor, peppermint and eucalyptus oil.

Uncle believed very strongly in the relationship between health and food. He said: "Ayurvedic medicine understands the properties of many foods and uses this knowledge daily. Turmeric is used as an antiseptic and can even rid you of poison in cases of snake or spider bite. Ginger and cardamom are used in improving blood circulation." Every household grew a *tulsi*, or basil plant, for effective relief of digestive problems, and for its use in religious ceremonies.

Uncle was a very religious person and read the Hindu scriptures daily. He fasted once every fortnight, taking no solid food for 12 hours. "It is good to give a rest to the digestive system," he said. I joined him in his lotus position for meditation, in his *prayanam* or breathing exercises, and in his fast. My uncle instilled in me that I should be very active, and showed me yoga *asanas* (postures). I could do most of them – but not, because of my injury, those which needed both arms to be used. Uncle showed me the "greeting the sun" asana which has twelve poses stretching the back and legs, then a press-up followed by steady standing on tip-toes to greet the sun.

I went and sat with my uncle in his shop and helped make herbal potions. I was known in the village as "the doctor's nephew". I exchanged *namaste* greetings with the boys, as we put our hands together as if to pray, and bowed our heads to touch the fingers. Everyone had a shower in the open space near their homes in the compound of the house. Drying after a shower was not a problem because of the heat. I put scented oil on my hair, and parted it on the left. I wanted to look like Dev Anand, an Indian actor in Bollywood films. Dev had flowing hair, parted on the left side and I thought he managed to look both very smart and romantic.

Auntie Indravati's food was usually dhal which had been cooked on a slow heat with butter added afterwards. I went to the *tandoorwalas* with the dough and saw at first-hand how to make tandoori roti. A *tandoor* is a large clay oven with a wide opening and a small opening at the bottom so that the wood fire could be lit and the ashes taken out afterwards. When the oven is hot enough, the dough is made into flat circles and put on the wall of the tandoor with a cloth-covered pad. The roti came out crisp on top and deliciously brown. It was smeared with butter, and I got it wrapped in a cloth and took it home. We had dhal, coriander, chutney, and onion salad sprinkled with lime juice.

One night we were treated to *kheer* (rice pudding) which was cooked slowly over 24 hours with a thickened layer over the top and with the addition of almond and cardamom. We had some digestive pills which my uncle had made in his dispensary. I think the ingredients were *amchoor*, mango powder, *ajuian*, black salt, honey and peppermint covered with an edible silver paper.

The following day I had a very interesting journey with my uncle to the next village, ten miles away. He had been asked to see a patient who was very ill and could not move. We were provided with a bullock cart as transport, and I rode the donkey (the first time I had done so). Someone helped me on and I held on to the donkey's mane to control it as there was no saddle and no reins. Our three-hour journey, which produced a lot of dust, was an adventure, as the donkey would sometimes gallop and sometimes refuse to move, or it would wander towards the fields and eat the greenery and drink from ponds, sometimes bending down so steeply that I found it difficult to hang on. If the donkey saw another one in a field or on the road, it made a sort of barking noise. On reaching the village, my uncle was greeted by the patient's family. We were taken to examine him, spending around two hours there. Uncle prescribed medication in the form of mixed herbs and inhalations. By burning specific plant leaves, a milky liquid was produced, and I was told that this was for breathlessness.

There is in Sardhana a very large cathedral established by a Muslim princess when she converted to Christianity. It has a convent school attached, and priests and nuns live there. I often visited this place, thus coming into contact with other religions.

Over the days of my stay in Sardhana I learned a great deal about village life and the *panchayat* system to settle disputes between village community leaders. *Panchayat* literally means assembly (*yat*) of five (*panch*) wise and respected elders, chosen and accepted by the village community. Traditionally, these assemblies settled disputes between individuals and villages. I have always remembered that one can achieve harmony by listening to the advice of others, and although I didn't take much notice of this at the time, it has left its mark on me. The whole holiday was a wonderful experience for me. When I left Sardhana, it was with regret that I could not stay longer.

So I returned home. But in fact I was not to be there for much longer.

15: Thapar Nagar

WE NEEDED A HOUSE with more room and some outdoor space once my youngest brother Ravi was born in 1951. There were eight in our family now and so we came to move to Thapar Nagar, still in Meerut.

We boys did not know what to make of Ravi, although I remember him as being very cute. He arrived mysteriously from nowhere and just simply came and took up residence with us.

Our sister Shashi was very attached to Ravi and carried him everywhere. We brothers inclined more to piggybacks, galloping wildly around whilst Ravi clung around our necks with his chubby arms. Ravi walking in the courtyard without a stitch of clothing is chiselled in my memory; I remember with amazement that he did not care what anybody thought of it. As he grew up, he always addressed me and my elder brothers as *bhabhaji* – "Elder brother, with respect."

Later on, when I was in medical school in Amritsar, once or twice a year I would have saved enough money to buy a train ticket home to Meerut. The train with its 20-or-so sleeper carriages steamed into Meerut Cantonment about 4.30 in the morning. I would then take a rickshaw along the wide leafy roads of the army cantonment, past the sleeping barrack huts, through the gates and into the tight little lanes of Meerut city. Early morning mist mingled with the hazy dust kicked up by the bullock carts on their way to the sugar refinery. The rising sun glowed red and shone on the tea vendor, coughing as he took down the shutters to his tea stall. At last we turned into the courtyard of my home. Silently I raised the latch and stepped into the dark interior. But Ravi was wide awake and waiting to jump into bed with me to hear all my news from medical school!

Thapar Nagar was a good place to live – a new colony. It was built on a grid system with nine lanes radiating from a big roundabout in the centre. It was a mixture of residential and commercial premises. Building work was still in progress in the area when we moved in, and there was a big hole in the ground where the builders dug out the mud to use in the construction, and piles of rubble stood everywhere.

We lived in a compound with seven other families, but *our* house was not new. Our main living area was one room and a small attached kitchen, both with corrugated tin roofs. The room was eight feet square with a window at the back, looking on to a large piece of waste ground. The roof was of asbestos and the window had shutters inside. We used this room to entertain visitors, and we children all studied in there at night when it was possible.

There was no electricity and lighting was by kerosene lamp. There were two communal lavatories, two washrooms and two hand pumps. The ground of the compound was not made up, and during the monsoon season it became a muddy quagmire. But all the children played there, whatever the weather. Because we had no storage space, Bauji went daily for supplies of fresh vegetables and groceries, and at the weekends I often went with him, enjoying the sight and earthy smells of all the fruit and vegetables. Beeji was always up before six in the morning, getting water for our bath or washing our faces in winter with hot water boiled on the coal fire. Father had already been to collect the milk from about two miles away – straight from the cow so he could be sure it was fresh and unadulterated.

Our breakfast was food left from the night before, usually dhal and *chapatti*. Sometimes, Beeji mixed dhal with flour and made *paratha* by gently frying the resultant pancake on the iron griddle over a coal fire. With this we had yoghurt, while the adults had pickles. Beeji made yoghurt every day, as this was the most nutritious food she could give us. The younger two had milk for breakfast and the rest of us had tea or sometimes half tea and half milk. A real treat was *double roti* (bread bought from the baker) toasted, with slightly salted butter and half a boiled egg, but this only happened when guests were staying or when Bauji and Beeji were feeling very well off.

One of my earliest memories in Thapar Nagar was of a huge, huffing, puffing, screaming and steaming, groaning, all-cogs-whirring, road-rolling engine. I was fascinated by it. There was a huge metal wheel with a large chain in it and a very large rear wheel. There was also a small green wheel near the driver, and it was always spinning. I always wanted to get on it, but never did. I loved the big whistle and used to walk in front of the roller so that the driver would hoot it to warn me and others to move out of the way. The roller was used to level the road surface as they made a new road with steaming black stuff. After the roller had gone over it, the men would sprinkle it with cold water which I could never understand. We all spent a lot of time watching this huge machine moving a small distance. We could certainly entertain ourselves in the street. I thought I was mechanically minded and got involved in watching *anything* being made.

There was a regular knife-sharpening wala who would go from gali to gali (what we called the narrow lanes) and we would follow him. I watched him make his wheel spin by moving the pedal, and I loved the noise made when sharpening the knife or scissors. Sparks flew all over the place and I thought they would burn our clothes or skin, but they never did. Once he had finished sharpening, he used a large leather belt to rub the cutting edge to make it smooth.

We ran all over during the day, either chasing each other, trying to catch an unclaimed kite or playing cricket. We would climb stairs or piles of rubble at a building site in the multi-storey buildings. We often fell and scraped a knee or an ankle. Because I never wanted Beeji or Bauji to know, I would cover the graze with spit and dry soil so that they would not stop my great adventures for fear it could cause a problem to my injured arm. This trick always worked for me. I have plenty of trophy scars on knees, ankles, arm and elbows to prove it.

Father's coal business was close to a run-down Muslim cemetery. My friends Rajesh, Kamlesh and me liked to explore this cemetery: we could usually find berries to eat and improve our aim at the squirrels with our catapult, *gulale*. We were discouraged by Muslim elders from wandering around in the cemetery ground but we did not take much notice. Not, that is, until a Muslim shopkeeper nearby told us that at dusk he had seen a mongoose biting the Achilles tendon of the corpses in the graveyard, causing the corpses to spring upright. The mongoose then dragged them off to its lair, so it could consume the dead flesh. We did not visit the cemetery again for a long time!

In summer we would have a quick shower outside near the hand pump, wearing only our shorts. After drying, we always used perfumed oil or Brylcreem to moisturise our hair, and for prickly heat we used talcum powder. Beeji would be ready with food. We would normally sit in the shade to have lunch together, usually one vegetable and yoghurt with maybe coriander chutney and chapatti and fruit in season. Our favourite was mango. Father would try to get some after finishing work. Sometimes we were treated to water melon, although yoghurt or milk products were not allowed with it, as the two curdle in the stomach.

The heat was overbearing and it was very, very difficult to rest in the house without electricity. Beeji and Bauji and some of the others stayed inside and had a siesta, using hand fans. Sometimes we would get branches from the khus khus plant to hang across the window, and then one of us would pour water on the leaves and branches. This gave us a cool breeze with an aromatic khus khus smell and was the air-conditioning of my childhood.

I spent a lot of my time in the afternoons visiting neighbours and school friends. I would try to find a house to visit, especially if they had an electric fan. We would spend time playing games. My friends were relatively better off than me and lived more comfortably. Sometimes I spent time at Father's third cousin's house, teaching the young girls mathematics and science – good practice for teaching in future years.

In the summer holidays all the boys were very keen to read *jasusi* (detective stories) and often would finish a novel in a couple of days. Some of us would try to read books in English – not easy, but considered by our group to be academic. These included such titles as *The Jungle Book* by Rudyard Kipling, *The Arabian Nights, The Serpent and the Rope* and *On the Ganga Ghat*. Later on I also read poetry by Ravindranath Tagore, *Feluda* by Satyajit Ray, and *The Good Earth* by Pearl S Buck.

In the evenings, about four or five o'clock, the family would have tea but I was always missing, playing cricket or kite-flying or riding with a friend on his bike. We were all interested in world cricket and knew of cricketers such as the Nawab of Pataudi and Colin Cowdrey from England, and we would go to great lengths to follow commentaries at the radio shop in town. I was fortunate in having a friend who had cricket gear, although I didn't have any myself. We sometimes used pieces of wood as bat and wickets, and played with a tennis ball. Meerut is well-known in India for its manufacture of sports equipment, but we could not afford to buy it.

In the evening we played the game of *kabadi*, a five-a-side game unique to Asia, with a playing area 20 metres square and divided into two. In the middle, a player from one side starts saying *kabadi* repeatedly and goes across the line to touch an opposing player without taking a breath. The object is not to be caught before getting back over the line and home. My friends in the neighbourhood included boys in the same year but at different schools, and we gelled well. We thought of ourselves as good singers, and as ten-and-eleven-year-olds, we sang patriotic songs together. We often put on performances for younger children, who looked up to us and applauded our every action!

After my arm operation, to keep myself occupied, I would often go with Bauji to the fruit and vegetable market. The market was colourful and deliciously aromatic. It is traditional to go there every day for fresh produce, picking the best and having it weighed, then bringing it home in a jute bag that we always carried, no pre-packed anything or plastic bags. I became good at recognising all the fruit and vegetables and enjoyed the whole market experience, meeting Bauji's friends and learning, from his example, to treat everyone with gentleness and respect.

Summertime in Thapar Nagar, when there was no pressure of studies and exams, was a happy time for me. In another way it was also very difficult, owing to the intense heat. Some of our neighbours' families went for holidays to Simla, Nainital or other cool hill stations. We never thought of it, as we knew that Bauji could not afford it. We were happy with our simple pleasures in life. In summertime, showering was easy – we went to the pump in the compound with a bucket and *lota* (jug) and red soap. I never had a bath in my childhood. Drying after a shower was also easy – we just stood around in the sun and were dry in no time. In the winter months a shower was difficult. Mother used to boil water on the coal fire and mix it with cold water. We would wash and then pour the water over our heads. Sometimes we could warm the water by putting a *balti* (large saucepan) of water in the sunshine for an hour or two.

I loved to go for an early morning walk during the long summer holidays. We would get up between four and five in the morning. At this hour it was not difficult to rise because the intense heat, even in the night, made everyone sleep very lightly. We often made straight for Company Bagh and the Meerut Military Cantonment. It was leafy and green there, and in the Military Cantonment the roads were straight and wide. We always walked at a brisk pace, expanding our chests with deep breathing and swinging our arms in military fashion, as we thought it was good for our health. We would reach the garden in no time and do our exercises. We greeted the sun, did press-ups and rotational body movements. Our Yoga *asanas,* the postures and breathing exercises we used to attain physical and mental control and tranquility. Hindus believe that yoga exercises unify the self with the Supreme Being.

And then I went running round the field. We would walk on the dew as it was believed to improve the eyesight! We would then make for the farmers' fields nearby to get some water from a well. The water, used to irrigate the crops, was brought up in small metal buckets on a wheel turned by a bullock. As we noticed the first rays of the sun, we would wash ourselves and we knew it was time to turn towards home, for breakfast. We usually got home about 6.30 to 7am, before it became hot.

During school holidays, breakfast was taken at a leisurely pace. Mother usually made parathas, stuffed with *dhal* from the previous day's meal. Sometimes she stuffed the paratha with cauliflower or spicy mashed potatoes. We ate them with yoghurt or mango pickle. When we were very young, we had milk to drink and, as we grew up, we drank masala tea – which is water, tea leaves, milk and sugar all boiled together in a saucepan. Families had their own variations of what spices made the perfect masala tea: our family used *saunf* (fennel) seeds, *elychee* (green cardamom) cloves and a sprinkle of pepper. If I was invited in by friends whose houses had electricity, my afternoons were spent in playing cards, snakes and ladders, carrom or monopoly. If we stayed at *my* house, we sat near the window to get the breeze, or we fanned ourselves with hand-held fans. This used up our time and sapped our energy. We perspired profusely and we could not settle down comfortably.

In the evenings I often went out exploring Thapar Nagar with my friends. There were large cultivated fields with carrots, *muli* (radishes) and cucumbers in our area and they were protected by a wall eight feet high. But we scaled the wall and stole the vegetables. We had to clean them by rubbing off the soil, and then ate them. Most times we got away, but on one occasion we were cornered by the farmer who was waiting for us on the other side of wall. He waved his stick and shouted at us and we knew the vegetable stealing game was over for good!

The ripening fruit on the trees was everywhere. We picked unripe mangoes, guavas, chikoo, papaya, *imli* (tamarind) and peaches, all without the owner's permission. These unripe fruit tasted delicious but often gave us the tummy ache we deserved.

There was a large *bail* tree near our compound, the fruit of which had a very hard shell. I often climbed the tree to shake the fruit off. Once, a fruit as big and heavy as a large coconut fell on my head. A large lump appeared on my head and I suffered headache and dizziness for a few days. I would not tell Beeji, as she would have been very concerned, then she would have been very angry.

Raj had left for engineering college and his bike became available. This gave me more freedom to go to the city. I became so skilled in riding the bike without holding the handlebars that I would show off. I would also free-wheel with the front wheel in the air and I found I could balance on a stationary bike for a long time.

These were the days of rationing. Wheat was provided as aid to India from America. We were given a set amount every month and sometimes I would take the wheat grain to the flour mill in town. The flour mill was very interesting. There were about three machines grinding the wheat, run by one motor with a belt to provide the necessary power. The wheat was tipped out on a platform five feet high, and grain was fed into a hopper above the grinding stones. The wheat was gradually ground into flour. The heat and wonderful aroma made me feel hungry.

We could not store much food in our house; so every time something was needed, we went to the market. In the summertime Beeji cooked vegetables or dhal in the evening, and sent one of us with dough to the tandoorwala nearby. A number of families had their tandoori roti made there. It only took two or three minutes to cook. Our tandoorwala would often amuse us by making the roti into different shapes. Sometimes he added onion or coriander for flavour. We all liked tandoori roti and Beeji was spared making it in the heat of high summer.

Chutney in our house was made by grinding onion, coriander and chillies, using two flat stones. Shashi could do this quite quickly without much trouble. We always had onion and lemon with our meal. Beeji liked *achars* (pickle) as she was very fond of spices. I often went to the outside kitchen where she would be cooking vegetables. I would pinch some half-cooked pieces. I was hungry and she would playfully slap my hand as she pretended to disapprove. This was my trademark in the kitchen and the family teased me. The habit has stayed with me all my life.

Most of my time was spent outside, walking and playing with friends in the neighbourhood. There was no space in which to play in our small house, but there was room to play on the street and this gave me the freedom to wander around, seeing some very interesting situations. Domestic animals lived all around us on the street. No-one kept animals as pets, so any dogs we saw were street dogs owned by no-one. They were fed by families, or they would walk into a house and help themselves to food. They slept on the pavements near food shops. I didn't understand when I saw male and female dogs joined at the back. One of our older friends explained about how puppies came to be born from this performance. It was a shock to me – that a dog couple would remain united for so long while we boys tried to separate them by throwing sticks as the two dogs ran side-step, still joined together.

It was normal to see cows all over the street. As they are sacred to Hindus, we knew that we could not cause them any harm. In the street they would eat any vegetables they wished. And if they felt like some shade on hot summer days, they would settle down anywhere, even in the middle of the road and stop the traffic. I liked watching chicks waddling after the mother hen. They were a beautiful yellow colour, and soft to the touch. I used to pick them up and feel their heartbeats and the sounds they made.

I loved going to market, the hustle and bustle, packed with food and people. Stalls and vendors spread out beyond the market areas. The ground spice stalls were very colourful, with bright yellow turmeric, fiery red chilli, warmly fragrant brown *garam masala* and khaki-coloured coriander, the powders in open jute sacks, piled high into cone shapes. The air was thick with strong aromas, as the spices were ground by the bucketful into the sacks.

We could not afford to buy fish or meat but I still liked to walk through on my way to the vegetable market. I could smell the meat before I saw it. Cages were packed beyond capacity with chickens and ducks. I could hear the sound of knives being sharpened. A man with a chicken draped over his bicycle handlebars passed by. I saw a family of partridges, their heads hung between the bars of their prison cage. Live cockerels and chickens were crammed into cages with other birds, such as pheasants, partridges and pigeons. I saw the butcher reach into a cage and grab a chicken. It squawked as he held its body between his knees, grasped its head and cut through its neck with a knife. He then twisted its neck and pulled its head off. I was really shocked; suddenly the chicken was free and headless, running down the street, blood spurting from its neck.

As I turned the corner, I found myself suddenly standing in front of a goat's head on a large metal plate. Its eyes stared blankly, seeing nothing. I have never forgotten seeing that and I didn't go near the meat market for weeks. We only bought meat when we had guests. I did have chicken once when my uncle visited. He was very fond of meat and poultry.

I ran errands for mother every day, usually when visitors put a demand on our kitchen that could not be met with the supplies we had. We could not afford to buy in bulk. Because we had no electricity, we had no way to keep things cold, so fresh produce was bought and used immediately. To get to the market, I ran through the area where lots of pigs were kept. Bright red piglets ran around my feet, squealing and getting in my way.

They rooted round and ate any rubbish and rotting vegetation on the road and in the drain. I amused myself by chasing the piglets to catch their tails. They were always too fast for me and I never did manage to catch one. They would squeal and shake their ears violently to ward me off. They could charge at you, which I thought funny at the time.

On Begum Bridge, over the *nala,* the large gully draining the town sewage, fortune tellers sat cross-legged, waiting for custom. They had a few trained birds in cages and a pack of fortune-telling cards. They would get a bird out of the cage to pick a card and then, from this, tell your fortune. They usually charged two or three *annas* a go, and usually predicted that you would become rich in the next year and would be successful in your job.

There were the monkey shows too. The monkey would beat a small drum and perform a trick or two, such as standing on one leg, or turn round and round, or sit on the shoulders of one of the thirty or forty people watching, and whisper in that person's ear. Sometimes the monkey strapped bells to his legs and danced.

On the road to Company Bagh there was a bear show which I sometimes stopped to watch. The owner held the bear with a chain fixed to a ring on its nose. The bear then performed for the crowd on his hind legs and turned round and round in time to a stringed musical instrument, while everyone clapped as he shook his head. Then his owner went round with a cap for contributions from the crowd. When the bear came to Begum Bridge crossroads, farmers up from the villages, balancing huge bundles of produce on their heads, stopped to see the show. Rickshawalas, schoolchildren and passers-by swelled the crowd. Bringing up the rear of the show was a couple of dusty elephants covered in red and green cloth, garlands of flowers swinging round their necks. Soon the traffic could not cross the bridge. Convoys of dusty lorries, a tractor or two and hundreds of bicycles were all held up in a noisy and chaotic jam.

I saw a lot of girls and boys going to and from school on rickshaws. They were small children, and the rickshaw owner would often place an extra plank of wood on the rear of the vehicle to provide seats for more. These youngsters, who attended Sofia School and St John's School, run by the nuns in Meerut Cantonment, were well dressed in their uniforms of brown skirt or short trousers with a dark blue shirt, and always looked happy. These schools charged the parents very high fees and I knew that I would never be able to get into them because of my parents' financial situation. It crossed my mind at that time that money was very important and that without it no-one could get an education or get on in life. But once the thought had passed, I was back to my world of kite-flying and other activities.

One day, on an errand to the market, I saw a lot of people gathered around someone who told fortunes, so I joined the crowd. The fortune-teller asked me to come forward, and told the crowd that I would tell the truth and the fortunes of all gathered there. He asked me to close my eyes and put in the palm of my hand a folded piece of paper tied with white string, and then asked me to close my palm. He told the crowd to ask me any question, for instance how many brothers they had, or were they married or not, and how successful they were in business. To my surprise, I answered all the questions correctly and the fortune-teller was able to sell the white paper tied in white thread for a small fortune.

Summer evenings were very hot and could remain hot until past midnight. As children we enjoyed it very much as we could play into the night. We were always late for the evening meal, which we finished quickly to get back to our games. In our compound of seven families, hide and seek was very popular. Sometimes we would play at catch-chase, and I was very good at dodging any chaser. Following the evening meal we would go for a walk to try and catch a breeze.

Sometimes we went to the main road to get paan. We would come back and make our bed on the charpoy. We would then look for shooting stars and count how many we had seen that night. On a full moon night, it was just like daylight. We would look up in the night sky to make up and tell stories of the different areas of the moon that we could see. The mosquitoes did not seem to bother us, although there were hundreds around, attracted by the open drains and stagnant water. There were neighbours who had mosquito nets which they draped over their charpoys. Our family did not have any nets and did not feel any the worse for it. I did not feel any poorer without all the modern facilities and we were happy with our lot.

After the intense heat of summer, we looked forward to the rainy season which arrived at the end of July or beginning of August. The sky turned yellow and the sun appeared a lavender colour. We could feel the rain in the sky but it would not fall. Suddenly clouds would appear in the sky; strong winds would whip up from the south and then would start the six-week continuous deluge! It all started with one or two big fat drops of rain. The drops rapidly became a torrent, hammering down on tin roofs and parched earth. Everyone came out to stand and enjoy a good soaking. Beeji would look up to the sky and say loudly: "God has come and given us great relief!" Fascinated by the accompanying thunder and lightning, I would go up on the roof to watch the lightning go from one side of the sky to the other – the bigger and bolder the better, as far as I was concerned. Not content with just watching it, I wanted to know where the end of lightning went, while Shashi was frightened of thunder and would hide under the divan or charpoy.

In the very hot weather preceding the monsoon season, we often suffered the intense itch of prickly heat rash; and now Beeji, knowing that this was the best cure, would encourage us to go outside, shirtless, in the strong pelting rain, splashing each other with water from the river or from puddles on the road. She always prepared good food on rainy days – masala tea and paratha with chutney, or she would give us a treat with *besan* (gram flour) omelette which was, she said, "heart-warming". And everything stopped when she made our favourite fried sweet pancakes with mango pickle.

During the monsoon we were trapped inside the house, amusing ourselves by playing cards, carrom, and snakes and ladders. I would read a great deal, finishing a book in one or two days. We became bored with the constant rain and hung our heads out of the first-floor windows, shouting for the *mungphaliwala* (peanut seller) on the street. We would lower a basket from the window, together with some annas and he would send the hot roasted peanuts up to us. Once the rain had stopped, there were plenty of puddles and the drains were full of dirty yellow-brown water. By evening we saw frogs hopping all over and they croaked all night. We stumbled all over them when walking in the dark.

I would chase and catch *jugnu* (glow-worms) with their tiny flashing lights like stars in the sky. Putting them under my shirt, I would take them home so that my younger brother and my sister could see them flying in the dark room, and would place them on a *chuni* (lady's scarf) and put it around my sister's neck, making her glow in the dark. Sometimes I put them under girls' blouses, thinking in my innocence that they would tickle and make them scream so that we boys could have a laugh. I put the glow-worms in a jar to keep them for the daylight and try to find how the light was produced.

16: New Neighbours

OUR NEIGHBOURS were varied. Near the gate of our compound was a Sikh couple who did not have children. They were very religious and attended every function in the *Gurdwara*, usually bringing prasad for all the children in the compound. Mr Singh wore saffron-coloured clothes during the day, as a sign of being an orthodox Sikh, and at night he dressed in military style to act as night security guard for our local colony. He would spend all night going round the houses, tapping his stick loudly on the street to ward off any intruders; he also had a large whistle to blow in case of problems.

Our other neighbours lived on the other side of the gate; they had two sons. Mohan Singh was a modern Sikh with short hair and no beard. Our two families were very close – he even referred to Mother as *Behanji* (sister). Beeji and Mohan Singh were forever cracking jokes. Practical jokes are well-loved in Punjabi communities. On one April Fool's Day Beeji invited Mohan Singh and his family round to our house. They had brought some *barfi* wrapped in silver paper. It was a hoax – dough covered with silver paper! We laughed and then we offered them some of our sweets. Their mouths began to foam, as our sweets were made from soap!

The third neighbour, Inder Lal, had three sons and two daughters. He ran a greengrocery stall in the market. The stall was dimly lit, cows and goats roamed through, eating vegetables that had dropped on the ground. Inder Lal was a scrawny man. His fluffy hair and beard made up for the lack of flesh around his face. He always greeted Bauji with a polite bow and *namaste*, good day. He would affectionately squeeze my cheeks and chuckle. I was puzzled by the beads of perspiration on his forehead even in winter, especially as he was so thin.

His eldest son Sunder was going to join the Indian army and was always keeping fit, using me and his younger brother as weights to build his arm muscles. He was big and tall. He had a luxuriant curly moustache which he constantly twirled between his fingers. Whilst waiting for his call-up into the Indian Army, Sunder kept fit by lifting 10-kilo sacks of wheat or picking up large stones to lift high above his head. He would invite me and his younger brother to sit, one in each of his arms and then slowly he would lift us into the air. He said that was a good exercise as he wanted to have equal strength in both arms. He developed his pectoral muscles to be so strong that he would invite us to hit him as hard we could, but he just grinned and swatted us away like flies. He could do a hundred press-ups without breaking out in perspiration. We often joined him in press-ups, jumping up and down and skipping with a rope hundreds of times.

The greengrocer's family was very religious, and the children went to the mandir every day. Frequently I went with them. One of them was my close friend and we always went to the Rama and Krishna. Here we took off our shoes, washed one hand and rushed to ring all the bells as we went inside, kneeling down in front of the statue and saying our prayers. On the way we were given crusted sugar sweets of flower petals as prasad. I was very intrigued by statues that could get me what I asked for in my prayers!

The neighbours on the right side of the compound were a couple who did not socialise and who kept to themselves. The husband was in the financial world, about which we knew nothing; and his wife was very particular about cleaning. I had never seen anything like it. Her face was always covered by her sari, which seemed to be washed hundreds of times every day. She had a ritual of first washing her hands in coal ash – sometimes a few times, sometimes ten – and then washing the pump spout and handle until shining clean. She was obsessive about cleaning her room and the surrounding part of the compound and was always suspicious of children because we made the place dirty.

We would often go to the pump and put coloured dye on the handle before she went to wash herself – amusing to us, but not to her. She knew very well it would be one of us boys in the compound but she could never catch us. When her hands were stained with dye, she would scream at the top of her voice: "Bagalfool! Stupid! and *Kutay ka beta! Son of a dog!*" and "Stop the boys using this pump!"

We had two pumps in the compound and she did approach Beeji and Bauji and the other parents to request children use the other pump at the far end of the compound. But nothing was ever done and we continued to torment her. As soon as we saw her near the pump, we would disappear round the corner and down the street but – to our delight – we could still hear her shouting and screaming.

There were families living in shacks along the road. They probably owned the pigs that ran in the streets – and I often saw as many as fifty to sixty piglets running free. A surprise to me was that the piglets were fed rubbish of all kinds but looked pink, clean and attractive. I don't know how.

On the other side of the road from our house there was a potter who moulded clay to make beautiful little devas and *gharras* (big clay water pots) for the shops. I was interested to see how he moulded *surahees*. These are elegant clay containers with a spout, used to keep water cool by evaporation in the summer heat. Another potter further down the road sat in the hot sun without shade or shelter. He only made the large clay gharras. He did not have any food or water with him. I wondered at the time how he survived and I wished I had some money to buy a gharra from him.

17: New School

THERE WAS A VARIETY OF SCHOOLS in Thapar Nagar, from the private convent fee-paying school to the municipally-run schools. We went to a council-run school where attendance was free. Our school was not known for over-achieving pupils. I knew that one could get into any institution with enough financial backing, but I also thought it was just not possible for me. It was a blessing in disguise because, realising that success in any field would have to come solely from my own efforts, I worked away and did my best.

The arm operation caused a lot of disruption to my study and I must have missed months of school. I began going with my friends to the local library where I read the newspapers, both local and English, learning about the world, science and the stars. I read English novels and exchanged ideas with anyone who would listen, trying to converse with them in English, and on occasion we would go to the local convent school to see an English play such as *The Importance of Being Earnest, The Comedy of Errors* or *Hamlet*. The plays were performed at a slow pace and the acting was real compared to Bollywood, where there is always overacting and the ending is always good over evil. I really enjoyed the plays and it was a very good introduction to English literature.

We brothers walked to school, three miles away in the city. We walked along and crossed the roads, elder brother helping younger. On arrival there was assembly, then in turn we shouted the times tables at the tops of our voices. This was repeated at the end of the school day, and within a few years we had learned the multiplication tables up to 19.

My earliest memory of writing in school was on a wooden board smeared with yellow clay which had been left to dry in the sun. This was my paper. I wrote with a small bamboo stick, sharpened at one end. I had an inkpot with ink, and in this way I learned the Hindi alphabet. As I grew older, the clay board was replaced by a slate in a wooden frame and a piece of chalk. We were taught both Indian and English history. We had very inspiring teachers who delved into many aspects of history. We learned of the ancient Dravidians who settled in the Indus valley in 3300-1300 BC, through the Mogul invasion from Persia and their mighty buildings including the Taj Mahal, to the British Raj and finally the formation of the biggest democracy in the world. We learned of the life of Mahatma Gandhi, his trial and imprisonment in South Africa, and the great Salt Marches in protest on the British tax on salt.

Generally there was a good atmosphere. Our teachers, although strict, were kind and caring. We had no playing fields, and sports time was spent in the school compound, clapping hands and climbing on each other's shoulders. During break times, we drank water from the pump and sometimes one of us would bring a bag of roasted peanuts for sharing. Some children brought food, maybe a paratha, some fruit and *lassi*. We would finish at 1pm and make our way home in the sweltering heat, walking in the shade of buildings and trees.

Our school taught us to be self-sufficient. We had classes in making cotton thread. Every town had a *khadi* shop and every spinner's efforts were sent to the shop. The school was asked to help the community by digging a canal about 15 miles away. It was to be a tributary of the Ganges, helping farmers irrigate their fields and orchards. We felt good about helping India become self-sufficient and make progress, and all Indian schools at that time were involved in such projects every month. Schooldays were full and enjoyable. There was a strong nationalistic fervour at the recent Independence of India. Slogans saying "Work hard to improve your life and prosper" were repeated again and again. Cinemas had movies with a self-sufficiency theme, and any ceremony in the community would be followed by the national anthem *Jana Gana Mana*.

There was very little space for a study room in our house; we had one room for five brothers and our sister. We had no textbooks of our own and often borrowed them from friends or at the library. We would copy important topics to study. I would go to the park, Company Bagh, and revise for my important exams under the beautiful bougainvilia tree. I have a memory of walking round and round the tree, repeating a list or table over and over again until I knew it by heart. For lunch we took some roti and pickle, or if I had some money (which I earned by teaching young children) I might buy some snacks near the park gate. Sometimes I would eat the unripe fruit dropped on the floor from the guava or mango tree. I must have spent hours in the Company Bagh when doing my matriculation and Intercollege examinations, and can still remember very well the places under the trees where I used to study.

The subjects in school were Hindi, English, Sanskrit, History, Geography, Maths, Chemistry, Physics and Biology. I would walk round and round the trees in the garden for hours, memorising every lesson till it became second nature. I cultivated a photographic memory and was able to reproduce texts without difficulty by associating various paragraphs with mango or guava trees. To help both me and our neighbours, I taught their younger children times tables and mental arithmetic. Sometimes for fun on full moon nights, I also taught the constellations of the stars.

18: New Business, New Pleasures

IN MY SUMMER VACATIONS, I tried to help Bauji in his coal business. He supplied coal to domestic and business customers. His labourers would use a wooden cart, pulled by a horse, for small loads and a truck for big supplies to businesses.
A few of Bauji's wagons delivered to the railway shunting yard at Meerut. The area was not secure. Stealing and pilfering from the goods wagons was constant. My job was to keep an eye on the wagons while Bauji was arranging coal to be delivered to the depot.

At the height of summer there was no shade in the railway shunting yard. The only way to get some shelter from the sun was by sitting under the railway wagons or their shadow. I spent so much time under and around the wagons that I became very familiar with all the undercarriage bolts and nuts. I learned that the train driver communicated with the guard through a tube connected under the wagons. During my stay at the shunting yard, I made a special effort to be friendly with the train drivers. One day my friendliness paid off, and I was invited up on the engine of an enormous locomotive. The driver showed me the intricate system of steam. It was mid-afternoon and very hot, but thrilling to see the engine moving and functioning. Pulling the chain to *toot-toot* the whistle was a dream come true.

I even had a romantic moment in the summer nights. I was playing near the house where I used to go to tutor the young children. I was invited by their elder sister to their roof-top, where she wanted to show off her knowledge of astronomy. I sat beside her and, with her hand on my shoulder, she pointed out the Plough and other stars. This progressed to holding my hand. She then scratched the palm of my hand. She said it meant that I was special. Before I knew it, she had her arms around my chest and she asked me for a tight squeeze. I hesitantly obliged. She had a strong jasmine perfume on her neck so I gave her a kiss on her neck and cheek. She got hold of me and covered me with kisses. I had never had any experience of this nature and I was overwhelmed. The meetings on the rooftop became regular, but we never met during the day. It was unheard of for a boy to meet a girl alone. Although she taught me about kissing and squeezing, I remained none the wiser about other things.

19: Snakes, Crows and Wasps

BIKE-RIDING OR WALKING, I would sometimes come across a snake charmer on the roadside. He would be playing a special tune on a flute – the kind of tune only played by a snake charmer!

Gradually, 30 or 40 people would gather round him to watch the show and I usually stayed to see it too. Then he would sit on the ground in a lotus position and, with ceremony, slowly put out three woven baskets beside him. He would start with a non-venomous snake, put it on his head and let some of the spectators put it around their necks or touch it. Next, he would show the fangs of a snake but hold its head and mouth open with a stick, and we would see the tongue suddenly flicking in and out of the snake's mouth. He would show us a double-headed snake, and I could not understand what it would eat or how it would excrete.

The highlight of the show was the opening of a basket with a cobra inside. A woven wicker basket lined with a khaki cloth was placed on the ground in the middle of the spectators. The basket had a closely fitted lid. The snake charmer skipped around, the bells on his anklets tinkling in rhythm to the strains of the flute. Slowly the lid of the basket wobbled and rose up, and the snake stuck its head out. The group of children held their breath as the snake slithered out of the basket. It moved its head gracefully from side to side as the snake charmer squatted before it. The charmer would tease the snake with his musical instrument, hit the top of the cobra's head with his fingers, and the cobra would try to bite his fingers or hand. The charmer always managed to avoid the snake bite and continue playing tunes on his special flute for a few minutes. This would mesmerise the cobra and it stayed in an upright posture and would go up and down with the movement of the flute.

The charmer would draw a mongoose from under his shirt. It would then become very active and, when the charmer put it up one sleeve, would crawl across his shirt down the other sleeve. He did a similar trick passing the mongoose through one of his trouser legs to the other. Our amazement knew no bounds

– we could not work out why the mongoose had not bitten him. I screamed along with the other youngsters in the crowd.

The next trick would be remarkable. He pushed a basket into the arena and started to play a flute. A corner of the basket would lift gradually and a young boy would appear from inside, even though the basket was impossibly small. The boy would produce a coil of white rope which uncoiled itself and rose eight feet into the air, and the boy climbed up the rope high above our heads. This, of course, is the famous Indian Rope trick. How is it done? I do not know. I can only tell what I saw. I am absolutely certain that the other spectators saw the same as I did. It will remain forever a mystery.

The whole show came to an end with the snake and the mongoose dancing beside the basket and then onto the charmer's shoulders. The charmer would then put his cap on the ground and ask for donations, and we would give a few *annas*.

Crows were everywhere in the towns and villages, picking over scraps of food and litter in the streets, and I regarded them as scavengers. Occasionally they would find their way into houses and courtyards and onto verandas, and they would congregate near food shops. I was not scared of them, but I didn't like them. And, if I got the chance, I would hit them with stones from my home-made catapult. I had seen crows in very large numbers in the park or at the gymkhana, where athletics and wrestling and cricket matches were held and which we passed on our way to school. One day there must have been thousands of them gathered there, keeping up a continuous cawing chorus. They would not stop even when I tried to disperse them with my catapult. I noticed that there was a dead crow in the middle of the throng, and later discovered from one of our schoolteachers that this was a crow's funeral procession that could last for days and days.

My friends and I stood with a group of villagers at the side of road, watching the crows. When a crow appeared to caw the sweeper's name, he was delighted and went away happy, saying it would bring him good luck. The crows were always fascinating. I had seen them looking for food, tossing rubbish into the air like ladies rummaging at a jumble sale. I saw a crow clasp a twig in its foot and sweep in the dust to look for grubs.

On another occasion I saw a crow fly up into the branches of a tree and drop a large nut from that great height to crack it. They jostled in mid-air and chased one another, "caw-aw-ah-ing" their loud throaty call and defending their territory from other birds. These sounds and sights were a constant background accompaniment to life outdoors.

I have never been scared of creepy crawlies; they have always fascinated me from as far back as I can remember. I was quite good at catching yellow wasps or big black ones by trapping them in paper. I would also take the sting out by pulling it, holding it with paper so that I would not get stung.

I would hold the wasp quite casually in my hand or hold it between finger and thumb and suddenly surprise my friends with it. I could provoke a bigger reaction from my sister and her girlfriends. I would amuse everyone by tying the legs of the wasp with fine cotton thread and let the wasp fly off, but of course it wouldn't fly very far! My sister told me that I was quite cruel and, much to my delight, her friends would scream.

20: Kuckoo is Injured

OUR FAMILY never lived in a house with electricity or piped water until after I had left home for university. We did most of the household chores and studying in the daytime, and in Thapar Nagar we studied in a small room by the light of a kerosene oil lamp which, very important to us, was meticulously maintained by Beeji, who trimmed the wick and polished and cleaned the glass thoroughly every day. The lamp had a steel base for the kerosene, and a complete conical dome which gave a brilliant yellow light. But mostly my studying was done outside, in the local park Company Bagh.

One day we were studying at home at the table by the light of the lamp. Kuckoo was studying for exams and wanted to concentrate, so he asked for time alone. I left the room and sat on the string bed in the courtyard. Kuckoo moved the lamp from the table and perched it on a cupboard ledge. I watched Kuckoo's shadow on the wall in the room, bent over the books. Suddenly he jumped up and screamed: "Fire! fire!"

I threw open the door and ran into the room. He was coughing and spluttering as I pulled him from the fire. He made a few choking sounds, then his legs buckled beneath him and he slumped to the floor

Bauji and Brij rushed in. Kuckoo's eyes peered from his blackened face. One side of his head smoked and smouldered as all his beautiful curly hair had been burnt away and we could see that his eyelashes and eyebrows had been singed off. It was Beeji who took control of the situation and lifted Kuckoo in her arms. She poured cold water on his burnt skin and yellow turmeric on his forehead and the raw skin on the side of his face, making him bright yellow. He was a real sight. Beeji consoled him, but I could see through the corner of my eyes that he was being very brave, biting his lip, and there were a few tears on his cheeks.

Bauji took the lamp outside and poured water on the burning wood ledge. That night Kuckoo slept with Bauji and Beeji. The rest of us lay awake for a long time.

As he began to recover, Kuckoo returned to sleeping with me. I told him that everything would heal up completely, although I had no basis for my statement. The incident left a mark on Kuckoo for some time to come, as he often woke with nightmares about the fire. He asked the barber to cut his hair very short so that he would not catch fire again. We teased him just as soon as we thought it was safe to do so.

We had another kerosene lamp too, which was used in the kitchen and out and about. Robustly made, it needed a strong hand to spring it open to light it; but once lit, it would remain so in the windiest weather – which was just as well, for we used it for walking on the street when shopping or visiting neighbours, and even when going to the toilet at night.

The kerosene lamps were very important to the family, and we all obtained good marks after studying by their light! I remember the smell of kerosene even now. And, as I start a garden bonfire with paraffin, memories of studying and laughter and family get-togethers in the light of the kerosene lamp come flooding back. But the traumatic experience with the lamp fire affected Kuckoo. He became very sensitive and introspective. He developed a weakness of his eyes and had to wear strong spectacles.

Beeji became very protective towards him. "Raj, if you've finished your homework, just go and sit with Kuckoo until he finishes his maths. He's got the lamp in there. He's still scared he'll knock it over." Beeji made sure both Kuckoo and the lamp were never again left alone.

The season of Holi and Dewali brought celebrations with fire, and added terror for Kuckoo. "I'll join you later!" he would say and we knew he would not turn up at all. The family were aware of his fear of fire and we stopped going to traditional firework displays.

21: Taking Chances

A GROUP OF US would often walk to the railway station with the intention of finding stationary goods trains, which we would then illegally board.

We would stand in the guard's carriage at the end of the train. If the guard was about, we would hide under the train, and when the coast was clear, we would climb on the guard cabin. Often we climbed up on the roof of the train so that we would not be caught by the guard. The train was often 15 or 20 carriages long; freight trains would be even longer. The carriages were pulled by enormous steam engines. With belching black smoke, hissing white steam and coal dust flying, the roof of a train was very exciting to us. Often coal dust would go in our eyes. We ducked and dived to avoid bridges, branches and smoke, and spread ourselves out flat when we saw an approaching tunnel up ahead. All this we thought great fun.

We were a close group of five friends, Kamlesh, Raj, Davinder, Lovedev and me. We would venture into sporty activities and often studied together as well.

Raj was the son of a businessman. Like me, he lived in Thapar Nagar, in the next lane to our house. Raj had a stutter and could never say words starting with K, S, or T. Sometimes it took him ages to complete a sentence. More often than not, much to his annoyance, we completed his sentences for him. We teased him and mimed the words he was trying so desperately to say. But if anyone else said even the least little thing about his stammer, we defended him, often backing up our disapproval at such insensitive behaviour with a punch or two!

Kamlesh lived very near to us and attended a private school. His vocabulary was, we thought, more sophisticated than ours; he called us "guys" and used English words like "goodbye, so long, see you later." Kamlesh had a squint. "How is one-eyed wonder today?" I always greeted him.

Lovedev was very proud of his name. He was always very keen to tell everyone that his parents had a love marriage so they named him Lovedev. He was also very religious and he attended daily prayers.

I was teased for my crooked elbow. It is known as a gunstock deformity, as the elbow is at the same angle as a broken shotgun and cannot be straightened. The elbow got in my friends' way when we were playing games. It often poked anyone near enough in the ribs. It worked to my advantage in sport, as no opponent could predict which way the ball, bat or shuttlecock would go. "Tell us which direction you are aiming at, Okhi!" they said, but I could always confuse the situation with my amazing arm!

We would wonder about in the lanes looking for things to do. We had got to the age when we whistled if we saw a beautiful girl in a tight dress. We often got a smile back.

In my childhood, telephone lines were provided by two cables on the street, to any number. In Meerut the houses were very close together with a narrow passage between the houses. These passages were only about six to eight feet wide in some places. Sometimes the telephone lines ran close to the window on the first floor and you could touch them by leaning from the roof or window.

One of my friends gave me his family's old handset as they were buying a new phone. I opened it up and found a round diaphragm which vibrated when you spoke. I decided to test it on the two lines which ran near the roof of my friend's house.

To my surprise, I could hear a constant buzzing noise from the phone and suddenly I could hear the conversation on the handset. My friends and I decided to bug all the conversations on the phone lines. We were pleased to learn about the mechanism of the phone although we could not make calls. We could repeat many a conversation word for word from the families whose phone we were tapping and we learned some very romantic secrets! I would tease older boys with the secrets I knew about their love affairs. They never did work out how I knew so much.

I connected my wires and listened. Crackling over the air came a Bollywood love song. I doubled up with glee as I recognised the melodious tones of Prem Bishnoi, one of our young neighbours. He crooned "Chaunvi ka chand ho" ("You look like a 14th day moon") or "Mere Mehboob" ("My Lover").

He spent ages serenading another close neighbour of ours, a young beautiful girl called Sushma.

One memorable day, I intercepted a call from the Gurdwara elders "That Mohan Singh, he's insulted us, himself and his faith!" they said, "Come on, let's get him!" Our compound neighbour, Mohan Singh, was a Sikh. He had cut his hair, going against one of the fundamental rules and outward signs of his religion. The elders at the Sikh Gurdwara had decided to take strong action. I flung the receiver down and ran to tell Beeji. She must have warned Mohan Singh, as within the hour his house was empty. The following day, five big bulky men, all elders from the Gurdwara, came looking for Mohan Singh. They had long white beards and wore royal blue kurta pyjamas and large turbans. The swords they brandished shone in the sun. They looked magnificent but very fierce. Mohan Singh went missing for a month. Beeji never asked how I knew and I never told her.

I learned new words and choice phrases on the line: "You filthy fornicator!" and "You son of a bitch!" and "You bastard, I'll make sure you disappear for good!"

But the most chilling was: "I'll drink your blood without spilling a drop!"

22: Intercollege

IN 1956, I PASSED my last school exam with good marks. I enrolled in the Nanak Chand Anglo Sanskrit (NAS) College to study botany, zoology, chemistry and physics. The College was about three miles from our house in Thapar Nagar and three of my friends and I walked there and back daily. We passed Raghunath Girls' College on our way to the NAS College. We would eye the girls, dressed in their blue and white saris or Punjabi suit uniforms. The girls remained distant until my sister Shashi, 18 months my junior, joined the girls' college. Suddenly I became very popular with my friends as Shashi and her girlfriends would walk with us to the college. I came to know my sister's girlfriends very well and I could introduce my friends to these mystery girls. They visited our house and I was called upon to escort them to the cinema or shopping.

In zoology I dissected cockroach's salivary glands, sheep's eyes, earthworms and rabbits. My rabbit specimen was considered good by my professor and was kept in the lab for reference for other students. Our main victims were frogs. We could dissect all the circulatory system, digestive and other systems. This was very interesting to young boys like me. We dissected on a wax table. First we had to catch our frog from the tank. We put a cloth soaked in chloroform on the frog's face till it stopped moving. When the frog was anaesthetised, we fixed it on its back and nailed it down with large pins on the hands and feet.

We would spend hours dissecting different systems and felt good about it in a curious way. I built a wax dissection table at home, and I would dissect frogs for their arterial, venous, digestive and urinary systems so that I could show my younger brothers, sisters and friends. I did not think that this was cruel but others did not like it. I always stitched the frog back up and released it back to the puddle. Some certainly survived, as we did see some frogs hopping about with cotton thread stitches protruding from the abdomen.

I wanted to do further practice at home. I stole a bottle of chloroform from college. The bottle had no cap, so I tied a rag cloth over and secured it with string. I put the bottle carefully in the top pocket of my shirt. Walking home, I saw a kite that had been cut from its thread coming down and I raced towards it, jumping over a wall to claim it. I bent over to pick up the kite and was overcome by the smell of chloroform as it spilled from the bottle and soaked my shirt. My friends following saw me disappear over the wall, but I did not reappear. They looked over the wall and saw that I had lost consciousness. They shook me to wake me up but I remained out cold for 15 minutes. The episode frightened me and I did not jump over any more walls with bottles of chloroform in my pocket!

Frogs were everywhere in the rainy seasons, in puddles near to the houses. Catching frogs became an art. I used paper to catch them, as they would always slip out of my hands onto my clothes because they had a slimy layer. Frogs croaked late into the night in the rainy season. We often stumbled over frogs in the dark and sometimes they were crushed. Baby frogs were particularly fascinating as they hopped and hopped, and were a challenge to catch. I would cup my hands and would keep the little frog in my pocket for frightening my family and friends, especially Shashi.

Some of my new friends had been to the Missionary Junior School where their lessons had been taught in English. They often spoke English at home and always in school. I joined the gang. The science studies at NAS College were also taught in English. We were interested in improving our English. We would go together to the main library and browse the daily newspapers, science magazines and world news, especially the English newspapers, to increase our general knowledge and to impress others with our spoken English.

We began to go to the Rivoli Cinema at 11am on a Sunday morning. We always saw English language pictures; epics such as Ben Hur, Cleopatra, Solomon and Sheba, and The Ten Commandments were our favourites. I thought that Hollywood actors had very expressive faces and moved their eyes and facial muscles much more than those in Indian cinema. I saw my first French kiss on screen and was very impressed with it.

We often went to espresso coffee bars to feel modern and think we were moving ahead in society. We would say "cheerio, so long, see you again and goodbye" without understanding the exact situation when these should be used. But we felt good. During conversations with my friends, I started using the word *chap* to describe anyone. I was using the *chap* word so much that my classmates nicknamed me "Chap". I have been Chap ever since; even now some my class fellows call me Chap instead of my real name. In college we had a close network of friends from different backgrounds. Devinder Chopra came from an army family, Rajesh Sharma was the son of a businessman who had a flour mill, and Lovedev came from a shopkeeper family.

In the Hindu religion, there is a system of castes. The Brahmin caste are holy men taking a pacifist and benevolent view of all creation; the warrior caste (*Khashatryias*) are dedicated to protecting the community and killing their enemies; and the merchant class have to do their best to see the community prospers. At the bottom of the pile are the scheduled castes: they are sweepers, cleaners and cobblers. Mahatma Gandhi re-named them *Harijans*, which means Children of God.

College was instrumental in bringing together young people whose paths would otherwise not have crossed. Not only did the differing social castes within Hinduism come together, but also Muslim and Hindu. And more liberally still, Muslim girls were educated alongside everyone else. These girls would arrive at college covered head to foot in their *burkha*. Once inside the classroom, they removed the outer covering and wore just a long dress and veil to cover the head. The caste system is less strict now and there is intermarrying between castes.

Studies were important as Intercollege exam results were essential for further university education. We were a group of six friends that studied together and exchanged notes. One of us would pick a particular topic and we would work together at college, after finishing at the end of the day. We would then make a presentation to the others, for them to examine and criticise. For us, it worked well and we all passed with very good marks. Some of my friends from other groups went to Engineering College and to further degrees in science and academic careers.

After two years of work we were getting ready for our Inter exams. During exams I studied in the park during the day and by the light of a kerosene oil lamp at night. Sometimes I would go to the house of my friend, who had electricity. Exams were held in the month of May when it is extremely hot. If I could sit under an electric fan, this was a real luxury. More often I would go and disappear among the greenery at the Company Bagh under my favourite trees – mango, guava, bouganvilia or neem – from morning till dark.

There were banyan trees, with large roots and a huge leafy canopy. Beneath a banyan the oxygen level is higher, due to the oxygen expelled by the leaves and roots, and the shade is very dense, as the leaves are many. I spent many hours revising my exam projects under the banyans – as Beeji said: "under the banyan tree one attains wisdom and fulfillment of wishes."

The hot pink blossoms of the bouganvilia, the red bottle brush flowers and the headily fragrant jasmine were very pleasant to sit under. Sometimes I would get under the mango or guava fruit tree; there I would steal the unripe fruits if the *mali* (gardener) was not watching. I watched squirrels scampering and jumping from one branch to another, either chasing one another or nibbling at the fruits. Noisy flocks of green parrots chattered shrilly whilst they bit holes in guavas, mangoes and peaches.

Exams were always traumatic. Luckily Bauji and Beeji were used to exams, as one or other of us children was always taking exams. Beeji developed an exam routine for herself. She gave us a head massage the evening before an exam, to increase the circulation to the brain, and also make us feel relaxed. In the morning she got up at four. She lit the coal stove and boiled the water for a bath. By the time she woke whichever of us was taking an exam that day, the tub was ready with lukewarm water. The bath was taken whilst sitting on a low stool and pouring water on the head. Then we would do our final revision for an hour. Beeji would be ready with a paratha accompanied by plain yoghurt and we were given a glass of milk to improve the memory. We had to eat soaked *baddam* (almond) which Beeji thought was excellent for a good memory. On my exam day I was ready to go to the college with my set of pens and pencils. I had Brylcreem on my hair and a splash of Bauji's after-shave on

113

my face. Exams were spread over two weeks. As soon as exams were finished, I was back to kite-flying, cricket, carrom or kanchan, and hide-and-seek on the moonlit balmy hot nights.

During the summer holiday I frequently went to Surat Ganj. This is a lake near Meerut Crematorium. We would go for a swim in the lake even though it was dirty and full of algae. It was here that I learned to swim. Beeji was very protective of me as I had had a number of mishaps in childhood. My arm operation made her determined to keep an eye on my activities. The more she tried, the more focused I became to try all the normal boyhood games and activities. I went swimming, climbing trees or jumping fences.

Beeji came to know that I was going swimming regularly. She confiscated my swimming trunks, but I borrowed from my friends. She went on confiscating trunks until she had built up quite a store. I think she had a real collection by the time I left for university.

"No you're not getting those trunks back! How many times I have told you not to go swimming? You'll hurt yourself on your elbow and infection will set in again!" she would shout at top of her voice. I would say: "Oh please, Beeji, I didn't go deep. I just went waist high. If you take my swimming trunks away, I'll swim naked then!" In fact, we often swam with nothing on, so no trunks was no deterrent.

The results of the Inter exams are very important and whole communities anticipated good results for their families and their friends. The results are printed in the main newspapers which arrive at Meerut city railway station. At this time, our family was not doing very well, with Bauji's business not as successful as it could have been, my own problems with my arm, and my older brother struggling to stay in further education because of a lack of funds.

"Please God, when is this is going to end?" Beeji would say with folded hands, looking up to the sky, "Maybe we have not done good deeds in our previous life. But still we do not deserve all this. Please guide us at this difficult time."

"Let us do something about it rather than talk," Bauji would respond.

Beeji wanted some answers – to know what could be done to improve the situation – and I went with her and Father to see Sadhu Ji, a fortune-teller. We went by tonga to the tiny *juggi* hut, which was home to the *sadhu*. He lived in the narrow winding streets of Meerut near the city railway station. He was dressed in the clothing of the holy man and sat in a hut made of mud brick covered in cow dung with, on the walls, a number of painted gods surrounded by *deva* lights. The juggi was very small, dark and had no window or ventilation. Incense and scented sticks burned their purple smoke; and on the bare earthen floor, in the middle of the shack, stood a three-legged table. In the corner was an alcove with an earthenware lamp with a wick made out of rolled cotton and filled with mustard oil. There was a flickering light casting long, quivering shadows on the wall. A thick layer of black soot covered the wall just above the alcove.

I felt uncomfortable in the tiny, dark and claustrophobic room, the strong smell of the mustard oil, and the dancing shadows on the wall. But most of all, I felt uncomfortable with the sadhu. I whispered to Mother: "Do we have to be here?"

She whispered back: "I've had enough bad luck to last me a lifetime, I'll do anything to break this evil spell."

The sadhu invited us to sit around the three-legged table and explained the process of how he would tell our fortunes. He asked simple questions about how many brothers and sisters there were, and their ages. Answers came from an unseen force knocking on one of the table's three legs. Bauji and Beeji seemed quite happy with this, but I felt uneasy about the whole thing and could not see how the knocking could just happen.

I asked the fortune teller about my exam results and he said I would just scrape through. In the event, I achieved a first class honours in the Intercollege finals! My younger brother Kuckoo went to the railway station and brought the news about my excellent marks. There were congratulations from family, friends and neighbours. Then there was a discussion in the house about my continuing education.

"You boys..." Beeji said, gesturing towards my elder brothers, Brij and Raj, "...want to do engineering. So Okhi, you should do medicine."

I protested: "But I have very good marks in maths, I would be better in engineering."

She took no notice. "No, you're very interested in medicine because you spent a lot of time in the hospital with your arm and you would make a good doctor."

Brij and Raj also thought I should take a medical path, so in the end I agreed to apply for medicine. Beeji was thrilled and shouted: "Professor Roaf will be proud of you! You become a surgeon, like him!"

I knew that Bauji could not afford the fees and I could not see myself in medical school. My elder brother was at university and the younger ones were at different stages of college. I decided to do a BSc degree in Zoology, which is allied to medicine as it is a science of animals. I had no offer of medical college admission at that time so I reasoned I could pursue a career in the Zoology academic department at Meerut College.

23: Milk and Bread

WE ALWAYS WENT to the farm for fresh, warm, creamy milk as Bauji felt it could not be pure unless collected from the place where the cows were milked. Normally he would go himself, taking a small stainless steel milk churn; but during the summer vacation I would take over to give him a break.

Mr Ahmed had five or six cows. As he knew our family and I was his youngest customer, he would show me how it was done and let me try. First he would rub the udder, then squeeze out some milk and rub the udder again, and to amuse me he would squirt milk straight from the udder into my mouth and down my face as well, saying that rubbing milk into the skin is good. Mr Ahmed's son stood in the corner of the barn feeding large leaves and fresh corn into a hand-operated chopping machine. There were other customers to collect the milk in churns and they carried the churns on their bicycle handle bars. Outside, cocks crowed and hens pecked in the barnyard and I would amuse myself by chasing the hens. Sometimes newly-hatched yellow chicks would be running in groups with the mother hen. I would catch one, look into its eye and feel its warmth and its heartbeat.

Milk is a very important part of a Hindu's diet, as it comes from our sacred cows. Milk is expensive, and poorer families – such as we were – gave milk at breakfast only to the very young ones or children doing exams at school.

We were friendly with the family who owned the King Bakery. The bakery was on the main thoroughfare. We would go there to get some biscuits baked. Biscuits in packets were very expensive.

The bakery was entered directly from the street through a low, narrow doorway. Once inside there was darkness and it took a few minutes to adjust to the low light. Three clay ovens were going at full tilt, with roaring fires beneath them. The flames flicked and leaped and the heat was intense. The walls were blackened by greasy smoke and the earth floor was covered in flour dust and broken biscuits. Mother asked me to take ghee, flour, sugar and some nuts to the bakery. The baker mixed the ingredients together and shaped the biscuits using his special cutters. Three bakers were on the floor, wearing vests and cloths wound round their heads to act as pads for carrying trays of cakes. They wore no shoes.

The trays went into the ovens on long-handled shovels and re-emerged ten minutes later as perfect golden biscuits. The whole operation was enjoyable to watch and made me feel hungry. Once I had to go upstairs, where there was a little landing with a door at the far end. Flour was being hauled up in jute sacks. There was very little light from the window at the end of the room, but there was a dim electric light over a long table where a man was at work skilfully decorating cakes with butter-cream and red and green sugar syrup. There were boys a little older than me who appeared very happy in their work. They laughed and slapped one another in friendship as they mixed and baked the biscuits and cakes. "How is my Patang Baaz?" one of them said, as they knew I was interested in kite flying.

"Come and join me on Sunday, you would enjoy it," I invited him.

"Have you seen Mere Mehboob? It is a love film with great songs and dances." He was obviously keen to talk. "We will go in few weeks time when the price of tickets has come down."

I felt quite easy talking to them as my friends and they often gave me broken biscuits and pieces of pastry.

24: Almost Drowned!

WE HAD ONE BIKE in the family, which really belonged to Brij. Cycling is an adventure to every child and we were no exception. My friends and I used to try stunts while sitting on the handlebars or back-wheel. Four of us could ride on my brother's bike and we would speed-ride, hands-free. This used to amuse my sister and younger brothers.

We could cycle to Sardhana village about 15 miles away. We would hitch a ride from a sugar lorry by holding on to the long stems of sugar cane sticking out from the back of it. We would take a picnic of roti and pickle. On the way we would stop at the Ganga Canal and the others would swim to cool themselves. I was officially barred by Beeji from swimming because of my fractured arm.

During one of our picnics, I dived into the canal from the high bridge, showing off to my friends. My dive was deep and I plunged under the algae. As I tried to surface, I could not see any bright sunshine or even daylight. I could not break through to the surface as I had been sucked under a large tree branch covered with rotting black leaves and stringy green algae. The strings of algae wound themselves round my arms and legs, holding me under.

Minutes ticked by as I kicked and flailed in desperation. I was trapped and my lungs were bursting. Frantically, I tried diving deeper, and finally I found a strong current, free of the tangling layer of vegetation, through which I could see sunlight. I surfaced, coughing and spluttering, about 300 metres further on, in the middle of the canal. Kamlesh and Lovedev were on one river bank and Raj and Davinder were on the other bank, shouting and screaming: "Okhi! Okhi is alive!" They were frantically wringing their hands and crying.

I was exhausted and shocked. I did not have the strength to swim to either bank because the current was too strong. They were barking instructions to catch the dead tree branches which they held out from either bank. With one last superhuman effort, I grabbed a branch and I was hauled out of the river by Kamlesh and Lovedev. They dragged me up the bank and on to the grass. I was covered all over in algae and dead leaves. Piles of algae had wound around my head as if I have been crowned. I was sputtering and coughing as I had inhaled lots of dirty water. They rolled me on my side. I was feeling cold and shivered uncontrollably. My friends stripped off their shirts and covered me. A farmhand on the bridge, who was watching the scene, gave Lovedev a blanket.

"We thought you are a goner! You've been under the water for ages!" said Kamlesh, "I was going to give you mouth-to-mouth resuscitation!"

"Over my dead body!" I retorted.

My friends had been scared to death and confessed that they did not know how they would break the news to my parents if I had drowned. I could not tell how long I had been under water and even now, after a lifetime, I cannot explain how I survived the ordeal. I rested for a long time with my friends around and we decided that I should travel back home on the bus. The others made their way back on bike and Lovedev brought my bike back by holding on to it while riding his own.

I came home with dry algae on my head and had a hard time explaining to Beeji my version of what had happened. I walked home from the bus station, which was about 750 yards from our house, still feeling cold and in shock.

When Beeji heard the front door bang, she vigorously tapped a spoon on the side of a saucepan in the kitchen area and came rushing through to the room with a face like thunder. "You've been missing the whole day!" she roared, "What have you been up to? What's that in your head? You look a real sight!" I hung my head and shivered; Beeji softened and looked concerned. She raked through my hair, muttering about how she never got a moment's peace.

"I slipped and fell down into the Surat Kunj Lake and I got stuck under loads of algae and leaves, I couldn't get out. I haven't washed my head properly," I whispered.

I think she knew there was a lot more to the story than that. She had an idea that I had been fooling around, but she also saw that I was very shaken and shocked, so she asked no more. She brought me a hot comforting chai and a blanket. Later she ordered me to get under the pump and got to work with the soap.

That night I had nightmares: I was drowning, tangled and bound hand and foot by strings of black and slimy green water weed. I was sucked down faster and faster into a black vortex, to which there was no end. The same nightmare came back regularly to haunt me for several months. I did not go swimming or diving for a long time.

25: Sugar Cane Fields

FATHER'S SECOND COUSIN was Dr Keval Chabra, who was a medical officer at the largest sugar factory in northern India. He lived at Daurala in a sprawling but basic brick house. The interior was dark and cool, shaded by wide verandas. The garden was lush and green; birds flitted in the large orchard containing guava, mango, pineapple and lichee. The house and garden were entirely surrounded by sugar fields. We could hear the thup-dup, thup-dup of water being brought by mechanical pumps into the fields.

We were fascinated by the gushing of water from the pump. We had a drink and washed our faces. My friend Kamlesh said: "Look! A chicken coop!" There were baby chicks all over, waddling in every direction. I was keen to catch a chick but, in spite of my best efforts, I was not successful.

My uncle gave us leave to go into the sugarcane fields. . We entered the cane field and promptly lost ourselves – the sugar cane was so tall that we lost our bearings. We walked between the rows and lay down in the crop, looking up at the blue sky. One of the workers cut the cane for us with his scythe whilst we peeled it with our teeth and chewed it to crush the juice out. Our hands and mouths became sticky and we enjoyed washing under the huge water pipe. Uncle then took me – along with my friends Kamlesh, Devinder and Raj – to the sugar factory.

In a corner we saw sugarcane juice boiling and thickening. At the other end of the room we saw sugar coming from the vat. We could not believe our eyes: the amount of sugar, the large piles of toffee, wrapped sweets, peppermints and lemon balls.

"Take some, take as much you like!" Uncle said. We gorged ourselves on lovely, sticky sweets. Then we became sick.

"Meri ma! Serves me right, my belly hurts!" Kamesh said under his breath as Uncle was nearby.

"Yeah, but let's grab a handful of sweets for later, when we feel better!" Devinder insisted.

In the end we became so sick that we did not bring *any* sweets home. Again, I got into trouble at home for not letting

Bauji and Beeji know that I had gone visiting. We got back again by hitching a ride on a goods train.

On the way back we could have ended up anywhere, as we did not know whether the train was heading for Meerut or not. Fortunately for us, it was.

26: Meerut College

I WAS ACCEPTED BY MEERUT COLLEGE in 1958 and it was a whole new world to me. I was at last climbing the ladder. I was joining the elite, the educated, and I was very excited.

I was also very excited to hear that the college was co-educational. Science classes are usually full of boys but, as luck would have it, zoology class was almost half girls.

The first day in college was an introduction to our tutors, a tour of the classrooms and laboratories and a look at the facilities available. I enjoyed the lab work. We were to do the dissection of snails and earthworms. We worked together, helping each other, including the girls. In a matter of weeks, we felt close enough to call each other by first names, which I had never known before.

I was fascinated by a Muslim girl in the class. She was in *purdah*, completely covered from head to foot in a huge black veil whenever she left her home. Fortunately for my curiosity she took off her *burka* in the class. The lack of sunshine had kept her complexion fair, but that was all. Over a period of time, we boys started walking with the girls and escorting them home. Sometimes I shared a rickshaw with the girls.

We were always up to mischief and we decided to have some fun at the girls' expense. Most of the girls had beautiful long hair. I was persuaded by my friends to tie their hair with black jute string to the bench during the class. When they tried to get up at the end of the lesson, we had already left the classroom and were waiting round the corner to see the fun and commotion.

On another occasion, we had a love letter sent to one of my friends. We tied it with string and placed it on the floor under the chair where the girl sat. She reached down to pick it up and we tugged the thread and flicked it away. We had a great laugh at her expense.

Now my evenings and weekends gradually became occupied with college activities.

I had already joined the NCC (National Cadet Corps). This was military training for all boys. We had army uniforms with all the extras. I wanted to be part of the battalion in spite of my arm problem. We learned how to march in formation, attend parade in clean and polished uniform, punctually every Saturday afternoon. Often we would go for a five-mile hike with our kitbags on our backs. After parade we were given a banana or an orange for attending.

A year earlier, when I was 15 years old, it had been the tenth anniversary of India's Independence from the British Raj and also the centenary of the start of the struggle, the first War of Independence. A troop of mounted cavalry trotted through the main thoroughfare of Meerut, followed by a band playing patriotic tunes; and, bringing up the rear, 5,000 of us young boys and girls in our National Cadet Corps uniform. We gathered at the spot where it all started, where the first shot was fired by an Indian soldier (a *sepoy*), killing his British sergeant, on this very spot, marked by this very stone memorial, in Meerut Army Cantonment, in 1857. After that, a gathering from Meerut marched to Delhi in the footsteps of the sepoys. Before setting off on the 45-mile journey, the young marchers paused to garland local Freedom Fighters who had been imprisoned for challenging the British.

Young men and women had chanted the sepoy rallying cry as they marched along "Dilli Challo!"("To Delhi!") and "Inquailad Zindabad!" ("Long live the Revolution!")

The NCC was considered to be National Service and the family felt proud of me when I walked down the street in full uniform, including cap, to join the parade at college. I started playing badminton and it was particularly pleasant to play in the evenings, on the floodlit courts. Soon I became good enough to play on the college 'B' team and represented the college in matches.

I did not have any zoology books of my own, so I either took notes from friends in class or visited the library. I studied late into the night by the light of our kerosene lamp and spent a great deal of time in the library. I found it difficult to invite friends to my home to exchange notes as I lived in a compound with one-room accommodation. Therefore, we would meet on Begum Bridge and exchange notes and sometimes go for a snack on the street. In the winter months I spent much time in the library where I could exchange glances with the young girls I fancied. We were not allowed to walk with girls on the road, but I was privileged to be able to escort the female friends of my younger sister. My male friends made fun of me because the girls knew me well; at the same time my friends were curious to know all about these girls.

Kamlesh was very keen on Sapna, my sister Shashi's friend. "Tell Sapna," he whispered breathlessly, "she has a curvy figure and is beautiful; tell her Kamlesh has sent this message." He shoved me with his elbow as if to say: *Go tell her now.*

I stammered: "I can't say that. It'll embarrass her and all her friends!"

The boys teased me: "With your charm, Okhi, you could arrange a meeting with the girls at Begum Bridge and we could all go for an espresso coffee, what do you say?"

In the end, with or without my charm, I could not arrange a meeting with the girls as they were very scared of what their parents would say.

Meerut College Library was a large, round, redbrick building, with two floors housing the science, maths, engineering and law sections; all other sections were downstairs. There was also a large area with a table and chairs for studying. The furniture and bookcases were very old but solidly built. We had to go to the librarian for help to find a book, as there was no comprehensive catalogue. I became quite friendly with our librarian. She happened to be the older sister of a boy in my class. Occasionally she would allow me to take books out of the library on her ticket as normally it was not allowed to take text books out.

At the end of each academic year at Meerut College, we had a College Week with all sorts of activities – sports, music and athletics. I didn't participate in the jump event because of my arm operation but always took part in the badminton tournament, becoming quite good. My opponents thought I had an undue advantage: because my elbow was the wrong way round, they couldn't work out in which direction I was going to hit the shuttlecock. Our tournaments were on a floodlit court – wonderful on a balmy summer evening.

We had a full athletics field as well as hockey, cricket and table tennis tournaments. One evening we had an Urdu poetry competition and a debating society competition, and there were also individual and group musical contests.

The last 24 hours of College Week were a day and a night full of fun. One of my favourite competitions was the sack fight, a contest between two students sitting astride a very greasy pole over a pond filled with red, muddy water. The two contestants were each given a sack partially filled with something soft and bouncy. The idea was to take a swing at your opponent and knock him off the pole whilst maintaining your own balance. Wrapping the legs round the pole seemed to be the best method, as we were not allowed to touch it with our hands. I was good at this game because of my slight stature and good sense of balance, which helped me to duck and dive. Fat opponents who swung too hard fell into the water beneath.

The event took place on a very hot day in July, in the midday sun. It was always very popular and nearly every student turned up. It was fun to splash water all over and fall in it occasionally. Our friends had hose pipes ready to blast the contestants off their poles. The opposing team hit us with water filled balloons. We were already drenched and thoroughly soaked before we started the contest.

Mr Verma, the master of ceremonies, blew the whistle. I swung my sack half-heartedly at Rajesh, my opponent, as I was ready to miss his swing. He did not take the bait. My next sack swing was a full-blown attack and Rajesh lost his balance temporarily. He came back with a left-handed swing which scraped my face. There was cheering from the students with every swing, and shouts of "Get him! Get him!" We must have been on the pole for 20 minutes. In the end Rajesh become too violent with his sack swing and I was able to duck under the sack and he lost his balance and fell in the water, splashing everybody. I was the winner! Everybody hurled water jets and balloons on me, which I thoroughly enjoyed. I got a stainless steel trophy, which I treasured.

On the last evening there was a concert, the highlight of which was a few sketches featuring portrayals of the Dean and our professors. Our illustrious Dean and his staff were always invited, and sat in the front row taking it all in good part. We borrowed props and clothes, and entertained with sketches wildly exaggerating any idiosyncrasies and mannerisms we had noticed in our tutors throughout the year, recklessly finding something to say about everyone.

Mr Verma was professor of Chemistry. He wore a kurta and pyjama trousers. He always wore a white cap and took it off as he entered the classroom. As the cap came off, his black hairpiece would fall sideways, revealing his white hair underneath. Suppressing the laughter was agony.

In the class the Biology teacher was always very polite to girl students but loud and abrupt to boys. He dressed immaculately in his suit and tie. His blue-black hair seemed to have stained his skin at the sideboards. As he taught us, he constantly looked skywards as if he did not want to make eye contact.

But the strangest of our teachers was the Physics master. Unfortunately, he had a tic, which caused him to suddenly explode in a spasm of flailing arms and frantic hand-wringing. Strangely, it never occurred when he wanted to write on the blackboard. He had bottle-end glasses and never wore socks, summer or winter.

In the end we would have a lovely meal together and go forward to the next year.

27: Best Man

I WAS STILL at Meerut College when I was invited by my cousin Sunil to be the *samphalla* (best man) at his wedding. I travelled to his house in Jalandhar by train and tonga. His Mother was the widow of my uncle killed in Kamalia during the Partition of India. I represented my family at the marriage ceremony and enjoyed meeting all the members of the wider family in Jalandhar.

My cousin, very much involved with Sikhism, was a regular at the Gurdwara, so we made a visit there for a blessing on his marriage. We spent the time together discussing his bride-to-be and he told me it was a love match, not an arranged marriage. Sunil saw the girl in the Gurdwara and was smitten by her beauty, so he found out from friends where she lived. He saw her in the park and asked to escort her. She also liked him very much but was scared that somebody might see them together and inform the parents, so she refused the offer. They started meeting in the park with other friends who would leave the lovers alone. They kept their feelings for one another a secret from their parents for some considerable time.

Indian society frowns upon love before marriage and it is particularly damaging to a girl's reputation. She is considered fast, loose, worldly and not suitable for an arranged marriage.

Their relationship blossomed and, after a number of months, Sunil plucked up the courage and asked the community matchmaker lady to find out about the family. Eventually they had to let the situation be known; and, after the initial shock, the parents accepted the situation and marriage was arranged. The night before the wedding, there was a party for all the family, friends and neighbours – a great feast with meat dishes, kebabs, traditional Punjabi food, and whisky all round. Out of respect for our elders, we younger ones drank our whisky from a glass hidden in a brown paper bag.

On the day, my duty was to look after Sunil, and towards evening we went to change for the night's ceremonies. The ladies looked gorgeous and cheerful, with jewellery on necks, wrists and tied *panjams* (silver anklets) on ankles. I had a western-style woollen suit. The bridegroom wore a silk jacket and a silver-and-gold-trimmed red turban from which hung marigold garlands, like a flowery curtain in front of his face. He mounted a white horse and I walked along beside him.

The groom's party made its way towards the bride's house, incorporating a rice-throwing ceremony along the way. The streets were lit by the large gas lamps carried by servants hired for the day. A brass band wearing colourful livery gave us musical accompaniment while we danced our way along the streets. There were three *dhol* drummers in the front of the party to announce the arrival of the bridegroom. My aunt reluctantly joined in and danced with the other elders, and the children had a great time doing their own styles, some of them very good. I am not a great dancer but joined in the celebration with glee.

We arrived to find the bride's house decorated with pretty coloured electric lights. There was a meeting-and-greeting ceremony between the bride's and the groom's relatives, starting with the two fathers. As Sunil did not have a father, an uncle represented him, and then brothers and sisters joined the mêlée, meeting with embraces so enthusiastic that they were lifted clean off their feet, accompanied by lots of laughter. We were shown to the *chamiyana* (decorated marquee) where pride of place went to the bride and groom sitting on golden thrones decorated with flowers. As the groom's samphalla, I had a place of importance at his right. We settled down and had light refreshments and a cold drink, then fell to some serious socialising and getting to know our new relations on the bride's side.

There is a tradition that young girls from the bride's side tease the bridegroom, so Sunil's shoelaces were joined together by unseen hands and, as he tried to get up, he stumbled and fell to the ground, causing gales of laughter. This is the one occasion when young girls can eye up the young men and come and talk to them. My cousin Sunil said it should come as no surprise if they played tricks on me, as I was considered an eligible bachelor. Giggling, six young ladies advanced on me, tied my hands behind my back and put ice cubes down the back of my shirt. They piled flower petals on my head. As fast as I shook them off amid shrieks of laughter, they replaced them. I did not mind at all and enjoyed the tease. "Hey, Sat, you next for this marriage lark then?" Just to return the compliment, we played tricks on them too.

A great wedding feast, set out in a marquee on the lawn was served. We started with hot *samosas*, colourful salads and sauces. Then on to the rich and warmly spiced mutton, chicken and vegetable curries, bubbling away in their silver samovars, all served with silver ladles that lay alongside; then the breads, finger-burning hot from the clay ovens and rice heaped up in saffron-coloured mounds accompanied the curries; then the *kulfi* ice cream, covered with pistachio and almonds stood in little cone-shaped pyramids on chilled serving platters, just ready for the taking. Lastly, the rich, dark slices of carrot halva covered with wafer thin slivers of silver. We drank Coca Cola, imported from America, in small glass bottles.

When evening fell, a mist descended. The caterers brewed hot sweet tea flavoured with cardamom. We took our tea in little disposable clay pots. We walked around helping ourselves to nuts and paan. The elderly men retired to a corner of the lawn, lit hookah pipes and puffed away until the religious ceremonies began at midnight. The ceremonies took place with the bride and groom, symbolically tied together with a red cloth, circling the *havan* (sacred fire) seven times while the pundit read the ancient texts and solemnly blessed their union. Then the newly-married couple prepared to go to the groom's house. There was an emotional farewell from the bride's parents to their daughter, and the traditional tears and wailing from the bride as they departed.

We visited the newly wed couple the following day. The *daj*, or dowry, was set out and displayed in the courtyard of the groom's house. There were saris for the aunties and gold jewellery for the mother and sisters-in-law. I was given a silver mug and woollen suit length for my role as samphalla. In the afternoon I made my way to the railway station, took my bunk bed in the third class compartment and settled in for the night.

28: Haridwar and Rishikesh

MY FRIEND'S FATHER HAD DIED. They were close neighbours of ours and my friend was the eldest son in his family and important duties would fall to him to perform for his father's funeral. I decided to attend the ceremony to offer my support in my friend's time of grief.

Following Hindu tradition, he had his head completely shaved, as only after this purifying shaving has taken place can the eldest son light the funeral pyre. The body, tightly wrapped in a white sheet, was carried on the shoulders of sons and close male relatives. The women gathered in the dead man's house, with the widow and the men and boys following the shroud-covered body down the streets. They chanted: "*Ram nam satya hai, satya bolo, satya hai*!" ("The only truth is God's name. Speak truth for truth is!")

We made for the burning *ghat* at Surat Kunj, in Meerut. Burning ghats are areas on river banks and lake sides all over India, set aside for funeral ceremonies: an area of level ground, paved with large slabs of stone or marble, with sometimes a roof built over, then steps leading down to the water's edge. The most desirable places to be cremated are on the banks of the Ganges.

Surat Kunj (Sun Lake) had a ghat, and my friend had a funeral pyre built on the flagged area. The body was put down on the wood pyre amid chants and prayers. Rich families could use sandalwood or camphor wood, but people from my district could not afford to cremate their dead in such a way, and we used ordinary firewood from the shop. We sprinkled incense and perfumes and my friend took a torch to set the pyre aflame in several places as he walked round it. The pundit chanted from the Gita, the Hindu Holy Book. We asked peace for the departed.

As the fire took hold, the flames leapt high and licked around the body until it disappeared in a cloud of fragrant wood smoke. Suddenly a loud noise, an explosion, came from somewhere deep inside the funeral pyre. I was startled and frightened. An elderly neighbour saw the look of horror on my face and whispered to me that the dead man's head had exploded with the heat, thus releasing his soul to be free to go on to his next life. All stayed until the body was burnt.

On the third day the family returned to "gather the flowers". The wood and body had burnt themselves out – all that was left was bones and ashes. These were the "flowers" we had come to gather in a sacred jute bag to be kept safe in the temple until such time as we could commit the ashes to the river Ganges. Hindu deities, or *murtis*, glinted from their alcoves in the dark interior of the temple. There was Lord Shiva, Krishna, Hunuman the Monkey God, the black and terrifying Kali, and Ganesh the gentle elephant-headed God.

A week later I went with my neighbour and his family and friends to a place called Haridwar, in Uttar Pradesh on the banks of the Ganges, a hundred miles north of Meerut, to put the ashes into the flowing currents of the sacred river. We engaged the services of a pundit sitting on the river bank. He led us all in chanting the mantras. The sons of the family got into the water and put the ashes in the Ganges. Pilgrims immersed again and again in the water. They pinched their noses as they bobbed up and down with the repetition of each mantra .There was group of women washing clothes on the stones and spreading them to dry in the sunshine. There were young children having their first dip in the Ganges. The parents said prayers and sprinkled water over the child's head to anoint it. It is the custom that men and boys can swim as they can strip down to their underpants. Women and girls can only take a dip, as women must remain in their sari and the girls did not remove their dresses. The ladies were beautiful as they momentarily disappeared below the surface of the water and re- emerged, their saris of green, pink and yellow clinging to their curves.

As we came on the main street, there was a festival and the road was full of the Hindu faithful in a state of religious frenzy. Dancers and musicians in procession with a drummer beating out furious rhythms were making their way to the temple. All were singing *"Hare Krishna, Hare Rama"*. Cymbals crashed as the crowd worked themselves into a sweaty trance.

We went to the pilgrimage area and immersed ourselves in the sacred water. People were throwing titbits into the water, and we were surrounded by big fish who gulped down the food. These were carp, between one foot and two feet long. They were light brown with large red marks and big fins, very slippery to catch. They were very used to humans and showed no fear, darting here and there between swimmers. They were fed by the pilgrims. I was very impressed to see their eyes as they looked straight into mine. The fish swam all around us as we splashed in the water, touching our legs as they darted about. I decided to catch one and put my cupped hands into the water. As my hands reached under a fish, I lifted it to try and get it out of the water. Although I was able to get close to the fish, I could not catch it. The fish got annoyed and bit my big toe. It was the first time I knew of anyone being bitten by a fish! Everyone thought it hilarious. I ended up with a small cut on my toe but I enjoyed the experience on the whole. Everyone was amused but told me to leave well alone in future.

Hindus believe water from the Ganges is essential in reaching the ancestors, and some families keep such water, *Ganges Jal*, in their house to be given to family members on their deathbed. Haridwar attracts poor and rich who have come for absolution and seek to escape from the cycle of rebirth and enter Nirvana, as well as non-religious people who come for a day out.

As the sun set, soft singing of the ancient Vedic texts began all along the banks of the Ganges, people chanted *Aarti* for the evening. Aarti is prayer led by a guru and chanted and sung by everyone. The mantras praised God and asked for His blessing on the people of the world. The evening Arti also saw a large bonfire lit over on the opposite bank of the river. The regular pilgrims, who knew the words by heart, shook their heads from side to side, keeping time to the chants. They clashed their bells and cymbals in rhythm. As darkness fell, the chanting reached a climax and hundreds of little *divas* (tea lights) sailed in their tiny leafy boats down the river; tiny petitions of hope twinkled their way down the river carrying the supplications, fears and hopes of a thousand souls. The little boats bobbed and swirled precariously on the water and into oblivion.

Following the ceremony in Haridwar, we called in at Rishikesh on our way back home to Meerut. It took us about half an hour to get there. From a small mountain stream, the River Ganges suddenly widens and gathers force at Rishikesh. A hanging bridge known as the Laxshman Zula swings over the river there. Ashrams, peaceful places for a spiritual retreat, line both sides of the river. Retired people, whose role in their family had become that of the wise and respected elder, came and stayed in the ashrams, seeking peace, spiritual guidance, and blessings for their passage into the next stage of the great cycle of life. They had been working all their life and wanted liberation from the material world and wanted time to contemplate. They lived with very few possessions and spent most of their time practising yoga and meditation.

The pundit told us that, on the 13th day after death, the human soul leaves earth and ascends into the cosmos to become one with the great universal soul. This day is celebrated with a family feast.

29: National Cadet Corps

ALTHOUGH I HAD A MEDICAL HISTORY of surgery to my arm, I was pronounced fit for military service in 1958. This really pleased me, as I wanted to be one of the boys. I joined the National Cadet Corps in Meerut College and was provided with full khaki military uniform including boots. Every Sunday afternoon saw us on the College parade ground. We were supervised by a major in charge and some NCOs. We were instructed in army discipline, marching on parade, and radio communication. After each session we were each given one or two bananas and a drink of orange squash or cold water. We gradually improved and started carrying backpacks of around sixteen kilos on five-mile hikes to build stamina. Soon we were even handling rifles.

Once we had passed the theory examination, we were taken to the rifle range and shooting practice commenced with live ammunition – each of us supervised by an officer from the army and hitting the target at 1,000 metres. I scored very good marks and earned a prize. It was a proud tradition: National Cadet Corps was looked upon by family and friends as national service. We had one camp a year, held in a different location each time. One time we were asked to join the NCC group from Jabalpur in *Madhya Pradesh* (Middle Province). This was my first trip outside *Uttar Pradesh*, (Upper Province) away from Meerut. I looked forward to these outings because we as a family did not have any holidays!

We packed our rucksacks, starched and creased our uniforms, and our boots shone from constant rubbing with spit.

The day came and we were 200 students gathered in college with our belongings. We boarded a train at Meerut City Station, and settled into our reserved third class compartments with sleepers above our seats. We were bound for Jabalpur – a great experience for all of us, and particularly for me because it was my first long-distance rail journey since the exodus of my childhood. The enormous steam engine pulled away from the platform and sped off with a whistle to the shunting area where the engine driver collected a huge amount of water from a large overhead pipe. There was steam everywhere as the staff attached the engine to the train.

We could see a huge trail of black smoke streaming backwards in the sky as we stuck our heads through the window. The engine puffed white steam from time to time, accompanied by shrill noises. Our seats were wooden with no covering, but we didn't mind. The windows could be pulled down and had wooden shutters so that the breeze could blow through. There were even some windows which had glass! The only lighting was from dim bulbs in the middle of the train carriage. I was fascinated with the view, watching life near the railway line go by.

We could see village life, both in the distance and sometimes quite near the track. Wildlife scuttled and birds flew overhead. Young boys and girls collected the coke cinders that fell near the track as we sped by; and as evening fell and the sun went down, the sun's rays spread over the trees in a yellowish and red glow. We saw the shadow of the train with the smoke from the engine making silhouettes. The most magic moment was seeing the sun set and the moon rise together. But Nature was a side issue for us, although we enjoyed the experience. We were more interested in talking amongst ourselves and telling jokes about our commanding officers.

One officer, a professor in our college, was always so full of himself. He had a mop of hair which blew about in the breeze like actors in a Bollywood film. He punctuated his speech with expletives and usually added "you bloody fool" at the end of every command barked in our direction, because he imagined we were impressed by his military masculinity and efficiency, whereas the truth was we were fascinated by his hair, musing about how we would manage to stand to attention if the thatch became detached and sailed away on the wind over the parade ground.

We also had a Sikh senior officer who would strut about like a cockerel, twirling his moustache and stroking his beard. His language was unsophisticated and sounded as if he were continually angry. He would roar "Ussi, tussi, saddey, twhaddey!" meaning "Me, you, mine, yours!" We would repeat everything he said back to him with an added "Yes Sir!!" and wait for his reaction.

Darkness fell and we sped silently on, past the twinkling lights of a distant village. After dark we settled down for something to eat. It was an adventure for us all to be having a meal on a train, and we didn't have a care in the world. We all did the clearing up. We were encouraged to sing, in groups or solo, keeping the beat by banging a spoon on the wooden seat, but gradually we all tired and settled down for the night, making our beds on the sleepers above. As we gathered speed across the dark and silent Deccan plateau, jackals bayed to the moon and their howls carried far on the still night air. Owls glided by and twittered their halting, ghostly call. I pulled my head in from the window and climbed up to my bunk, covered myself with the blanket and, rocked by the gentle motion and the eternal clickety-clack of the wheels, I knew no more.

Dawn broke and a thin streak of gold appeared on the far eastern horizon. The early morning light crept over the sleeping land, and still we sped onwards towards Jabalpur. In the villages cockerels cried, donkeys brayed their complaints as they were loaded up with bricks, raw cotton or vegetables, and wild boars snorted as they sifted through the debris beside the track. As we pulled into stations, *languar* monkeys chattered and screamed as they swung from the station rooftops looking for any food inside or outside the carriages. Quick as a flash, they swung down, collected their stolen goods, and scampered away to eat in the safety of the rafters of the station platform. At dusk, hundreds of bats flitted across the beams of light beneath the station roofs. As we pulled out of the station, the pink and grey dusk gave way to the velvet blackness of the night again.

Third class Indian railway carriages usually have bars at the windows instead of glass, so a hot dusty breeze ventilated our carriage day and night. Passengers travelling third class are able to hang out of the window and enjoy being part of the countryside; being enveloped in the occasional puff of smoke and soot is all the more exciting when you are 16 years old. The first things I noticed in the early morning were a slight breeze and sun rays on my face. The train was travelling at quite a speed and there did not seem to be much activity in the fields.

After an hour, everyone was up and we heard a commotion outside the train. Surrounded by engine smoke, we had stopped at a large station with hawkers on the platform, selling boiled eggs, tea and toast. We had breakfast and noticed that the air was cooler and local folk had their faces covered by mufflers and caps. Some were smoking bidis.

It took two days to reach Jabalpur, where we were to camp near the town. We were trained to erect tents as dormitories and larger tents for activities and games. We did our stuff on the parade ground and settled down to the more serious business of making friends with the students from Jabalpur. In the evening there were games and competitions. We watched local boys performing dances and groups singing, and we ourselves held singing contests.

We were allowed to go sightseeing during our stay. We decided to hire bikes from a local shop and go to a place about 30 kilometres away. This was a new experience for us and we thought of a brilliant idea! We would hitch a ride on the tail of a lorry and be carried, together with our bikes, to our destination. We did it, as always, by holding on to the long sugar cane stalks that invariably stuck out at the back of the overloaded trucks. We waited for half an hour to find a suitable truck upon which to hitch our lift.

It was dangerous as we could neither anticipate potholes in the road nor predict when the driver would apply the brakes, and we were on high alert because of the danger of being hit by another vehicle overtaking the truck. The brilliant idea lost its charm as we travelled in a cloud of dust and petrol fumes from the exhaust pipe. Clinging with bare hands to the sugar cane stems for an hour, we arrived at our destination hot, aching, sweaty and thirsty, but we did not peddle the bike at all.

We made for Bhera ghat, a famous beauty spot with a wide river flowing through a gorge, with sides rising steeply from the rough water. We stopped at a group of stalls and wooden carts huddled together on the roadside selling fruit, and we bought guavas, mangoes and tangerines. We then moved on to the *dhaba* café. It was constructed on three sides of corrugated tin sheets; the fourth side was open to the road. The roof of the dhaba was made of a rope framework over which was laid sheets of cardboard and jute bags. An open fire burned at the entrance, upon which a cook was making chapattis. Inside, large copper pans of lentils and vegetables bubbled away on a hob made from clay and mud and heated by a wood-burning fire beneath. We pulled up a stool and sat at the wooden tables to await our meal, served in a disposable bowl made from leaves. No need for cutlery, as we ate by scooping the vegetables and lentils up in little mouthfuls with the fingers.

The marble rocks and white limestone cliffs rose high above the water of the Narmada River. We were keen to see the waterfall at the head of the gorge. We could hear the thunderous roar as the water crashed over the top and down into the turbulent river beneath. I approached a boatman paddling very long oars over the side of his rickety boat and asked "Fall ka kitna paisa?" ("How much is it to go to the fall?")

"Paunch rupee for ake!" Five rupees for one person! We bargained for fifteen rupees for the four of us, then took turns steering towards the waterfall, whilst the boatman rowed; eventually he stopped the boat at a safe distance and we saw the water before us, like smoke cascading down from on high until it disappeared in a cloud of water vapour into the raging river beneath. The roar blotted out all other sound and the air was fresh and exhilarating.

Bhera ghat was magical and we stayed all day. We saw the gorge turn red as the shadows lengthened. We had heard that the gleaming rocks have a magical effect, especially by moonlight, so we were thrilled as the moon rose and the cool, gentle light bounced off the white limestone and marble and glittered and shimmered on the surface of the Namada River running far below on the floor of the gorge. Reluctantly we made our way to the ghat, the riverbank, for the return journey which took us nearly two and a half hours. We were exhausted and put our bikes in the tent at the campsite and settled down in our tent dormitory. We returned our bikes the next day.

30: Gods and Holy Places

OUR FAMILY belongs to a branch of Hinduism known as Arya Samaj. We believe the cause of all true knowledge is God, the Highest Lord, who is the maker of all. Every Sunday morning we attended a *havan* at which we chanted hymns (*Vedic mantras*) praising Almighty God and asked for blessings for us who work hard and help others.

But there are lesser gods also involved. A havan is a sacred purifying ritual of sacrifice to Agni, the god of fire. We burned wood and twigs over which we poured ghee to set it alight in a rectangular pan and added a mixture of herbs. This is to purify and enrich the air. This ceremony is also performed on special occasions such as birth, marriage, special festivals and death, or entering a new house or an inauguration. After the ceremony we had Prasad. The Prasad was usually *suji* (semolina cooked with ghee and sugar) and the adults also had tea. Sometimes a learned preacher, a visiting Arya Samaji, would give a talk, usually on wisdom and how to achieve it. As children we were only interested in playing most of the time, although some of the words did rub off on us.

Beeji and Bauji were very interested in voluntary work and were among the first group of Arya Samaj volunteers to give their services in Thapar Nagar. One particular episode was an invitation to work as a volunteer in a local eye camp, about four miles away. It was run by Thapar Nagar's Inner Wheel. Father and Mother were involved, and I also volunteered. I was taken with my friend in a jeep to spend two days as a general helper. We looked after people who were having cataract operations, escorting and feeding them. We slept in a tent for the two nights with other young student volunteers.

When I passed my first year BSc in Zoology, gaining admission to the university of my choice, everybody was pleased for me. Bauji and Beeji arranged a havan ceremony in the Arya Samaj temple in Thapar Nagar. I was given a blessing from them and all my relations, friends and neighbours in our compound. It was a great feeling that I had achieved admission into a prestigious institution on my merits without having to ask for any financial help from anybody. I felt very humble and had a few tears in my eyes to see my family, relations and friends wishing me success.

On the subject of religion, I very much liked the Hindu god Ganesh because he is the god of Learning and I prayed to him just before my exams. The temple to Ganesh was near the vegetable market. I saw most shopkeepers visiting it before opening their shops. They usually kept a picture or statue of Ganesh in the corner of the shop. They would ask Ganesh's blessings by burning incense sticks before the little shrine. They placed marigold petals on a plate and said prayers, with circular movements of the plate around the picture of Ganesh, before taking any business decisions. Ganesh is considered the guardian of new businesses and continued success.

Ganesh has the head of an elephant and the body of a human. The reason for this is that Shiva and his divine consort Parvati had a son, whom they named Ganesh. During his father's absence, Ganesh would stand guard for his mother. One day Shiva arrived home and wanted to see Parvati. Not recognising his father, Ganesh refused him entry. Shiva became angry and cut his son's head off. Upon learning that Ganesh had been guarding his Mother from danger, Shiva was filled with remorse. In desperation, he sought to replace his son's head and bring him back to life. Shiva replaced Ganesh's head with the head of the nearest creature to hand, which was an elephant.

As a young boy I would often see people in the street wearing orange *kurta pyjamas or dhotis*. They had large red marks on their foreheads and shaven heads or very short hair, with a tuft of hair at the back. I learnt from friends that these were Jains, a religious sect of Hinduism. One day, out of the blue, I saw a man, a Jain, walking without any clothes at all. His mouth and nose were covered by a white muslin cloth, so that he did not inhale flying insects. He wore no sandals so he did not hurt any creatures in his path by stepping on them. Someone walked in front of him with a broom; he swept the road, so the holy man was sure he would not be stepping on any living creatures. It was a hot day but the blistering road didn't seem to bother him. He was accompanied by followers who chanted, clapped and rang tiny bells through the bazaar and along the street to the temple.

There were men and women prostrating themselves in front of him, asking for his blessings. He was an important pundit and considered very intelligent. There were lots of ladies walking with him. I could not understand why they were not embarrassed by his complete nakedness. I discovered he was a guru on a visit from the Jains' main temple. He was worshipped to the extent that women would take home fallen pubic hairs as a symbol of their faith in Jainism. This I found peculiar.

Also on the subject of religion, Dussehra is a Hindu festival celebrated in late October, which recalls the mighty cosmic battle between the good king Rama and the demon king Ravana. The ancient texts of the Ramayana relate how Rama governed a peaceful and beautiful land. Sita, his ever faithful wife, was always at his side. Sita is the role model for Hindu womanhood. The demon king Ravana abducted faithful Sita and took her to Sri Lanka, where he kept her a prisoner. To win Sita back, a battle of epic proportions began.

The festival lasts about ten days. The battle is re-enacted by little boys all over India every November. With wooden swords and shields, we helped Rama regain the lovely and virtuous Sita. We made a stage from sheets hung on bamboo sticks and lit by kerosene lamps. We did shadow shows and performed Rama killing Ravana, saving Sita and bringing her home. For a concluding act, we made big paper images of the demon king Ravana, filled them with *patakas* (fireworks) and set them on fire, to show the victory.

Three weeks after Dussehra, there is the festival of Diwali. This is The Festival of Lights. The victorious return of Rama and Sita is celebrated with hundreds of tiny lights, twinkling in every doorway, street corner and garden wall, to guide the couple home from Sri Lanka. Mother was very keen to get the house white-washed before Diwali and she always painted the front door. We were told to keep the door wide open so that Lakshmi, god of money, would come through the door on Diwali night. Because we did not have electricity, we used hundreds of oil lamps and candles. The oil lamps were made of clay with a cotton wick soaked in mustard oil, then lit and lined up along the rooftop and walls or in the alcoves all around the house.

The smoke from neighbouring rockets, Catherine wheels and Roman candles was so dense that we could not be sure if our own patakas had lit properly or not, until they too sprang into pops, bangs, flames and a frenzy of shooting stars. We children jumped, danced and laughed with delight. I then went with my friend Ramesh to the next alleyway to see *their* fireworks. I would even make my own patakas. I used a tin and made a hole in it. I spat on a special chemically-laden tablet and put it underneath the tin. As I lit a match in the tin, there was a huge explosion; the tin flew high in the air with a bang. This was my cheap home-made patakas.

I was in big trouble with my parents when, one year, I tied a long line of small fireworks to a dog's tail. When they exploded, the dog went berserk and ran frantically all over, frightening everybody. At the time we all thought it hilarious but it was very cruel to the dog.

After our special Diwali meal, we would go out to watch the organised fireworks display, then come home to start our own. To handle money on Diwali night was thought to bring good financial luck for the coming year and would entice Lakshmi, the goddess of wealth, into our home. Father brought new rupee coins home and, following tradition, we sat down to gamble and play cards. I was always quite successful in winning a few extra annas as pocket money.

The day after Diwali also has a special significance. It is a time when sisters remind brothers how much they love them. A little ceremony which involves the trying-on of a special bracelet around the brother's wrist is performed. The bracelet is known as a *tikka*. Sisters also mark brothers' foreheads with vermillion powder and press some rice grains on top, also as a sign of their sisterly love. All five of us gave our sister Shashi a big hug and some sweets. As we got older, the sweets were replaced by money for a new dress or shopping.

There is a large Hindu temple near Thapar Nagar. There are statues of Rama, Sita and Lakshman, but the main statue is of Hanuman, the Monkey god. Hunuman is a disciple and protector of Rama and Sita. As a boy, I wanted to be Hanuman. He is thought to be very strong and he performs miracles. Hanuman could move mountains and forests and fly them from place to place in no time. I adopted him as my god and he adopted me. Hanuman's statue was red with a monkey face and a human body. We went on Tuesdays to ring the bells and pray for strength and money.

During Dussehra festival we were all excited about Hanuman's bravery. I was told that when Rama's brother was badly wounded in Sri Lanka, fighting the Demon King Ravan, Hanuman flew to the sacred Himalayan mountain for life-saving herbs and plants. Hanuman could not decide which one to bring, so he lifted the whole mountain and carried it to Sri Lanka. Some of the herbs and plants dropped down and, it is said, that is how life-saving herbs and plants thrive in that particular southern part of India.

The first time I saw a Sikh I was fascinated by his long hair and beard; grown men also have long moustaches which they are always rolling and twisting. Two of our neighbours were Sikhs; and once a week, like girls, they would let their hair down and shampoo and comb it, spending just as much time on their hair as did the girls. Sometimes, as a conditioner, they would rub yoghurt on their hair and wash it later. As I grew older, I had a Sikh friend whom I came to know well. Some people thought Sikhs were not bright people, although I didn't think it was true. There were lots of jokes about them – my brother Kuckoo used to say that something happened to them at full noon and that in the heat of the sun they became confused. A standard prank was to ask a Sikh near mid-day "Has it struck twelve?" They would always reply: "For us it is always striking twelve". I used to tease my Sikh friends about their beards and long hair and then tell them a Sikh joke, always told in a thick Punjabi accent with a rustic lingo. They took our silly jokes in good heart.

Near our house on the main road was a Gurdwara, a place of worship for Sikhs, very spacious and clean, run by volunteers and open every day to all people from different religions – particularly Hindus as their religion is closer in tradition to the Sikhs. As a Hindu, I often attended functions there in celebration of the birthdays of Guru Nanak Deva and Guru Govind Singh. Guru Nanak Deva was the founder of Sikhism in the 15th century. He believed it was not religion that determined the merits of a person, but his actions in the eyes of God. Guru Govind Singh was the tenth guru, who established a community of saintly soldiers. They serve the Sikh religion and are distinguished by their lovely blue uniform. They are known as *khalsa*, which means pure.

He introduced five symbols so that Sikhs can recognise each other. The symbols are known as the five *kakkars*. They are *keshar*, hair left uncut; *kunga*, a comb worn in the hair; *kachha*, underpants or shorts; *kara*, a steel bracelet; and *kirtipan*, or small sword, carried at all times. Because Sikhs never cut their hair, they wear it in a bun, covered by a turban. When we went to the Gurdwara, we took off our shoes at the entrance and covered our heads with a handkerchief. We saw very tall Sikhs dressed in blue clothing and smart turbans, their beards and moustaches properly folded. They wore their shiny kirpans. They were getting ready for a procession in which they walked in front of Granth Sahib, the holy book of the Sikh, four of them carrying the book on a cushion on their shoulders. Afterwards we all went into the Gurdwara and sat on the floor for *langer*, a lengthy meal – spicy *daal* made from a mix of several types of pulses, served with tandoori roti, salad and pickle, followed by *halwa* (sweet dessert) for the adults and fruit for the children. It was all donated and cooked by volunteers.

In summer we would spend much time in the Gurdwara, with Sikh friends from our compound, as it was cool and had fans going all the time. I liked the philosophy of the Sikhs – they teach that if you have done wrong, you should first try to put it right and also do some volunteer work in the Gurdawara and maybe make a donation, so that you have then made amends and are free to progress further to have peace of mind, to keep God in your heart and mind all the time.

In February, the day before Holi, Sikhs celebrate Baisakhi, by lighting bonfires, to mark the coming of spring. My friends and I attended celebrations all over Meerut. Everyone was dressed in colourful clothes. A group of young men in multicolour shirts and wearing fantastic turbans did a very strong athletic dance to the beat of *dholki* drums and rhythm sticks .We were all encouraged to join in the Bhangra dance, and some dancers lifted us young boys on their shoulders. Others were dancing with colourful hankies, rhythmic movements of the hand, shaking of the hips and body on half-bent knees. The whole atmosphere was electric. Lighted cinders from the bonfire rose into the dark sky like glowworms. There were *channa* and *puris* to eat and masala tea to drink. We would stay around late into the night and come home tired and settle into bed. The next day was Holi.

Some Hindus think the Holi festival is devoted to Krishna, Hinduism's playful God. I always enjoyed Holi because the festivities are centered on fun and mischief. Holi is celebrated in February or March with the flinging, throwing or squirting of coloured water at unsuspecting passers-by. At Holi, people wear their oldest white clothes. I would prepare myself for days before, getting out my large *pichkari* (water pistol) and looking for some powdered paint. We started squirting coloured water one or two days earlier on anyone passing through the narrow lane. We were hidden well away out of sight on the roof, so that we could direct streams on to the folk below.

On the day of Holi we would have our coloured powder and water all mixed up in a bucket. We started with family members, squirting the *gulaal* on Beeji and Bauji, then brothers and sister, during much laughing and hugging. I liked red and blue powders and I made a good pattern on my face. Then we visited our neighbours and friends, covering them with powder or sprinkling them with coloured water. The more reluctant the person, the more they were pursued. We even got a chance to touch the girls, who would scream at the sight of the dry powder being thrown at them. This was also the time to forget all past disputes and arguments and renew friendships between friends and neighbours. The spring festival celebration meal was roasted and blackened chickpea, prepared on the fire the night before. My particular mischief was to have a bucket of coloured water on the top ledge of the door: when a person went through the door, the water in the bucket would drop all over them. I enjoyed the fun.

It all finished by lunch-time and we would bathe and change into clean clothes and eat our meal. Special sweets were then passed around, bought for the occasion. Beeji was always full of fun and up to the day. She would make *bhang barfi* (hashish scones) and give some to everyone – family members, friends and visitors. The scones made us all sleepy and hungry. Beeji usually pretended to be high from eating bhang barfi as she swayed from side to side. All the ladies in the neighbourhood laughed and clapped at Beeji's convincing performance. We would bring out the *dholki* and harmonium and there would be a song and dance session. This was one time in the year when I saw my parents dancing together. Beeji danced as if she was intoxicated but we knew she was totally sober. Ramesh, Kamlesh and I drank *bam bam bole*, intoxicating liquor made from hashish. We shouted "We are Shiva's followers!" as we swayed all over the place. Lord Shiva, who spent a great deal of his time off his rocker on bhang, is the god of destruction and reproduction.

Because I was interested in other religions, my Father introduced me to Mr Massey, a Catholic Anglo-Indian. Mr Massey had a large family and they invited me on a shooting trip to an orchard twenty miles from Meerut. I was amazed to see so many different fruit trees in the orchard. There were three varieties of mango, limes, pomegranate, avocado, custard apple, plantain and jackfruit with its enormous green fruit, weird objects the size of a football with a delicately patterned rind. There were *chicoos* that looked like large eggs – chicoos taste fantastic, like fibrous honey; they have a glossy stone as if someone had polished it. There was a rose apple tree which really tasted of roses.

The orchard of mango, guava, papaya and bair trees was surrounded by a sugar cane plantation. We went in his jeep with two of his boys, Matthew and Luke, both older than me. I was given an air rifle and shown in detail how to use it. We were to shoot rabbit, pigeon and partridge; I had some success with pigeon and started trying for rabbit. But, although I must have fired eight or ten shots, the rabbit would always get away.

After a while I saw one standing still, even when I approached it, so I put my gun on the ground and tried to grab hold of the animal. To my astonishment, as soon as I stretched my hand in its direction, it vigorously scratched my hand and forearm with its claws and ran away. Mr Massey explained that you must always hold a rabbit by its ears – otherwise it would give you trouble. "Rabbits are very quick and you must lift it up in the air, otherwise you will either lose it, or, if you do get it, it will scratch you. I am sure you can do it." Mr Massey whispered into my ear, as he did not want to make any noise that might disturb the birds and other animals. Later I found the rabbit dead, so Mr Massey must have shot it properly.

Mr Massey said: "You boys get up in the *machan*, (hunting tree house) and you will be able to see the animals and birds in the trees." He patted me on my back. We went up there and watched the parrots eating fruits. Nestling in the high branches were also pigeon, partridge and peacock. Squirrels scampered all over the trees, eating fruits and nuts. We were amazed to see all the activities in the tree canopy. We watched carefully and quietly. Matthew and Luke were used to handling air guns. They were good shots and had bagged quite a few pigeons and partridge. We had a wonderful view and enjoyed the peace for an hour up in the machan. After spending the whole day in the orchard, we had around thirty pigeons, three rabbits and some partridge, and we sat for a picnic under the shade of a mango tree. Mrs Massey had prepared puri and channa and we took fruit from the orchard for dessert.

From early childhood, I loved eating large green round guavas when they were hard. Mr Massey collected ripe and aromatic guavas for making *chaat*. We peeled the guava and then cut them into pieces in a ceramic container and added salt, pepper, ground roasted cumin seeds, chilli powder, lime juice and little bit of sugar, and we ate it with toothpicks.

While we were enjoying our picnic, we suddenly heard a sharp sound from the orchard behind us, turned round and saw two peacocks walking side by side, not scared of us at all, as this was their home territory. For the first time, I saw a peacock display, the male making a great show of opening his colourful shining feathers, and Mr Massey explained that the peacock was trying to impress his mate, the hen. When they had moved away, I picked up some of the male's beautiful feathers, and brought them home. The next day Mr Massey brought delicious pigeon curry for our family and there were no pellets in it! I still have in my home today a rabbit skin which Mr Massey had cleaned and cured as a souvenir of my day's shooting.

I would visit St John's Anglican Church in Meerut Cantonment, where most of the worshippers were Anglo-Indian. I liked the Roman Catholic Church on the Great Trunk Road in Meerut, particularly at Christmas. I also visited the Cathedral in Sardhana when I was on holidays with my uncle. Because Mr Massey was a Catholic, he introduced me to the basic beliefs of Christianity. We had a very good discussion. We agreed that there is an almighty God and there are different incarnations in different religions and most religions preach peace, harmony and love for your neighbour. "But I cannot understand the virgin birth," I said.

"There are certain things one cannot explain in scientific terms and you either accept or reject it." Mr Massey was forthright in his thoughts, but gave no explanation.

31: Tongas and Rickshaws

BEGUM BRIDGE, dividing Meerut City from Meerut Military Cantonment, was a hive of activity and the place to find hundreds of rickshaws and tongas for hire. I would stop on the Bridge to see the activities. The tongawala shouted at the top of his voice the names of the villages to which he could take passengers, while his horses made snorting noises into nose bags made of woven reeds.

The horses, large plumes on their heads and clouds of hot air coming out of their nostrils and mouths, were fed fodder made with greenery from the fields. I loved the sight and smell of the greenery, freshly chopped by the hand-driven chopper. Sometimes the horses were restless, whinnying, stamping and swishing their tails.

"Patience, patience, we won't be long," Kundan, our tongawala, would say and he would tie the reins to the telegraph pole nearby.

"No horse is like *my* horse, look at the sheen of his coat, soon you will see him flying!" Kundan would leap down to take a villager's bag and say politely: "Sir, you take the front seat; we will leave very, very soon, just one more passenger."

Sometimes the man would not let go his bag. He would say: "What is the point? We are maybe an hour waiting for another passenger!" He would walk off and look towards a rickshaw on the other side of the road. The man would strike a bargain and jump into the rickshaw. Kundan would then say some choice words under his breath.

In the winter months the air at Begum Bridge was filled with smoke from fires lit in old oil drums. The rickshawalas and tongawalas would huddle round the red hot smoking oil drums, especially at night, to keep warm; and their heads and faces were swathed in shawls against the cold night air. Some of them would be smoking bidis; inhaling deeply in one long pull, they could smoke away half of one, exhaling through the nostrils, clouds of smoke swirling around them. They fascinated me by making smoke rings. I was tempted to smoke, but watching the tongawalas making explosive coughing bouts and lots of spitting and spluttering put me off. There was a wooden shed in which the older tongawalahs and rickshawalas always congregated, smoking hookah pipes with loud bubbling noises. There was lots of smoke rising from the shed and the smell of tobacco too.

I learned a few choice words describing men and women. Fights between tongawalas and rickshawalas over passengers often broke out. Tempers would flair. "Mind your words, you bloody fool!" And "You son of a bitch!" And "You'll pay for stealing my passenger!" To get the ladies, they used words like a dutiful son "*Mataji*, (mother) I will take care of you." And to the young girls in their colourful costumes came the flowery language: "You are the most beautiful girl I have ever seen!" There were five people already in a tonga one day, and this one was supposed to carry eight passengers. There was a family of six who wanted to go to Meerut Cantonment Railway Station – so, without more ado, eleven managed to squeeze aboard.

There were also hawkers near the tongawalas who sold hot roast peanuts. I remember one particular person call Nandu whom I saw all my childhood in that area. He was dressed in a dhoti and was always unshaven with a rolled-up moustache and a dirty green turban and was always in a bent-over posture. Nandu shouted with his typically low voice every time he saw somebody. I always felt sorry for him and I would buy some if I had enough money in my pocket. As far as I can remember, we always went by tonga or rickshaw to the Nauchanti Mela, which was held in Meerut every year, five minutes from the town centre.

It is a big mela incorporating an agricultural and business show, and I remember a great atmosphere with plenty of excitement for the children. There were chaat and paan shops and restaurants selling a great variety of food. There would have been ice cream too, but, as we could not afford it, we had crushed ice with bright red or green syrup poured over it. There were hundreds of side shows and hand-driven rides, and always a large circus. There were single-wheel bikes ridden by groups of girls and boys, and trapeze artists, and the show included tigers, lions, elephants, monkeys and bears.

Loudspeakers crackled into life announcing the show. Hawkers yelled their wares to tempt the customers in.

Motorbikes roared around the arena. The shooting gallery nearby occasionally rang out with as a volley of shots hit the metal targets. I was fascinated by a motor cycle which sped round and round and also up and down inside a wooden building. I could not understand how the rider could drive a motorbike on a side-wall inside this wooden structure. There was always a very large searchlight shining into the sky, rotating wildly, so that everyone knew the circus was in town. I remember going there every year in my childhood. Although we usually went to the show by tonga or rickshaw, we almost always returned home on foot.

32: Grandfather's Visit

GRANDFATHER was a tall bespectacled man. He wore the typical *salwar kamiz* and turban of a proud man of the Punjab. He visited us with a large basket of fruit. Beeji wore her sari covering her face that day, out of respect and modesty. She bent to touch his feet, which is the tradition. We children touched his feet but were lifted by him and given a squeezy hug which he said was the best thing in his life.

Beeji made special food for him. Normally for the family we had a vegetable dish, daal and chapattis; but for grandfather mother cooked two vegetables, a meat dish, daal, pilau rice and tandoori roti. There was salad and other pickles and poppadoms. Nearby Sadar Bazaar was famous for the Indian sweet *gulab jamun* and this was especially brought from there.

After dinner grandfather would take us for a walk. We usually stopped for paan on our way. He told us stories of his farming days and how he would ride round his lands on horseback to supervise the tenant farms. Grandfather's lands were so extensive he would be gone for three days or more.

Grandfather still had some land in the Punjab. It had been part of a compensation deal that had been forced on him in the dark days of Partition. He escaped to India as a refugee, and tried to start again. The land that was offered to him was not fertile and was one tenth of the acreage.

Grandfather talked to my elder brother Brij, and asked if he would be interested in farming the new land. Grandfather even suggested that he would buy Brij a tractor. Brij was halfway through a degree in Economics at the time. He knew the land would be unproductive, and so he politely declined.

Grandfather took a keen interest in our education. Being mindful of the gunstock deformity of my elbow and the operation on my arm, he asked me for which university course I was going to apply. He wanted me to go into medicine so that I could help others. He knew how Professor Roaf had changed my life. He said: "Congratulations, your Father said you achieved very good marks and won a scholarship, well done! I'm certain you'd make a good doctor!" Grandfather put his arm around me and gave a tight squeeze. I replied: "I'm applying for Glancy Medical College. I really hope I get it."

Glancy Medical College in Amritsar, together with the Medical College in Bombay, was the most prestigious in all India. At that time, just after Independence, there were only five medical colleges in the whole of India. Glancy received 5,000 applicants each year. "With your marks and scholarship, you'll get a place in the medical college. I'm so sure! I'll come and visit you in Amritsar. Your arm looks fine. Professor Roaf has given you a gift, a second chance. Go and become a surgeon and you will make Professor Roaf proud of you."

I said: "I'll have a go. Hopefully, one day I might make a doctor, God willing."

33: Medical College

I FINISHED MY ZOOLOGY COURSE at Meerut College a year early because I *did* win admission to Medical College in Amritsar in 1959. In that year, there were very few medical schools serving the whole of the Indian sub-continent, so the standard was high and the competition was fierce. The results of my Intercollege examination had won me the scholarship. I had no money to pay tuition fees so I would have to continue to gain top marks each year for the next five years, in order to retain the scholarship and qualify as a medical doctor.

There was a ceremony of havan before my departure and I had a blessing from my Bauji and Beeji and all the relations and neighbours in the compound. I went by train to Amritsar and took a rickshaw to medical college and settled into Block A. This was the first time I had been away from Meerut and my family.

The Medical College tradition of ragging the new entrants was both interesting and alarming. Two nights before the college was to open, we first-year students were asked by senior students, particularly second-years, to assemble in Block A Compound at dusk. There was a lot of commotion in the compound and then suddenly the lights went out. A very loud voice came over the public address system: "Get into the middle of the compound and take all your clothes off! Hurry!" We were all very shy and reluctant to take our clothes off but the voice in the darkness spoke again: "Hurry up, or we'll come and do it for you!" Thus threatened, we complied. "Stand behind one another and shout: *We look silly, we look silly!*" We did so. "Now," continued the voice "file past us, like the parade of silly fools that you are!"

We paraded three times round the perimeter of the Block. Torch lights flashed at us and a garden hose was turned on, sprinkling us at intervals with cold water. The initiation ordeal lasted for two hours. The ceremony ended when our chanting became tedious and the sight of our shivering naked bodies brought no more laughter. Next morning we again met in the compound. The ring-leaders who had organized the initiation introduced themselves. "You chaps stood up brilliantly to everything we dished out!" they said, "You've proved worthy enough and daft enough to be here." They all agreed: "You've joined the club now. We've been there last year. If you need any help with studies, anything you don't understand, we're happy to help." The senior students became our friends. This was a great introduction to college and a way to get to know the seniors.

Some of our seniors were a little bolder about embarrassing young entrants to medical college. They took the first-year students to the anatomy dissection hall where the cadavers were laid out on the tables, covered by a sheet. They had lit the place with flickering candlelight. The new students were given sweets and instructed to put a sweet in the hand of each corpse. A senior student hid beneath one of the dissection tables with the dead body above. The sweet was put into the corpse's hand. But as the new student turned to go, another hand thrust up from under the table and a loud voice demanded: "Where's *my* sweet?" The poor unfortunate victim was so shocked, he collapsed.

We first year students shared Block A with the second year. I shared a large room with three other new boys. There was a bed in each of the four corners of the room. We each had a cupboard for clothes and a table and chair for study. There was a large ceiling fan in the middle of the room. This was the first time I had used electricity for a light to study and to cool myself with an electric fan. The washing facilities were down the corridor

I did not have a bicycle in my first year. Anywhere visiting, we walked or took a rickshaw or tonga. We studied six days a week and attended lectures and did dissection in anatomy and experiments for physiological function of the body in the lab.

We started mixing and making friends. Our first year started in earnest with the study of anatomy, physiology and hygiene. Most of us had never seen a dead body lying on a marble table. We dissected for anatomical studies. I was curious to know where the medical school got the bodies. In fact, they were given to the college by the police authorities who had shot these smugglers on the India/Pakistan borders. They were all well-built male bodies. Red formalin had been injected to preserve the cadavers and to show different tissues clearly.

Formalin has a very strong and unpleasant odour. After finishing the session, we would wash our hands thoroughly but the stink still clung to our hands and clothes. I felt nauseous with the smell, but soon got used to the idea that first-year medical students waft a cloud of noxious odours behind them as they walk along.

We shared the dead bodies with the second-year students who were doing dissection of head, neck, abdomen and pelvis. We were doing the upper and lower limbs. Anatomy dissection tutorials were always in the morning. We were given proper white coats and gloves and we had our own dissection set of knives and forceps. As soon as we had finished, we went for lunch.

Food at the college was proper Punjabi: filling and plentiful. A lunch or dinner consisted of three dishes: meat, vegetable and lentil curries, accompanied by salad and roti breads. We were all assigned a helper who brought our meal from the kitchen, washed our clothes or ran to the dry cleaner, made our bed and polished our shoes.

My helper's name was Balbir Singh. He had many years experience in looking after young men at the college and away from home. I had great difficulty eating anything to start with, due to the stink of formalin and the thought of the dissection room. For the first month, I felt home-sick but Balbir Singh would say: "C'mon, keep your strength up, you've an exam tomorrow!" or "You'll see things differently in the morning!" In this way Balbir Singh helped me settle in to my new surroundings. I had biscuits and sweets from home, which I kept in a tin and opened whenever I felt home-sick or hungry.

Eventually I got used to being away from home and made many friends, some from such far-flung places as Malaysia and Kenya. The majority of staff and a great many of the students in the college were Punjabi Sikhs.

Amritsar contains the most sacred Golden Temple, headquarters of the Sikh faith. I had many Sikh friends in our compound back home at Thapar Nagar and my best friend as a boy was a Sikh.

The college was a co-educational institution and a quarter of the students were girls. The girls' accommodation was separate from ours, so we only met the girls at the dissection table. Traditionally on Saturday night, I went to the cinema with friends. Usually we went to the late show, 9pm to 12 midnight. We then walked home, feeling hungry. We would cook up fried eggs with green chillies on toast, covered with plenty of tomato sauce. On Sunday a group of us would go to town. We bought our essentials: perfumed soap, talcum powder, Brylcreem, shaving cream and Gillette blades. We would stop off for roadside snacks, sometimes golguppa, another time chaat and maybe some hot sweet jelabies.

In the evening we played games. My favourite was badminton, which we played on floodlit courts. After games, we were back to studies. I used to go to bed early, between 11 and 11.30pm, and get up 4am for study. Lectures and tutorials were from 6am until 1pm, Monday to Saturday. The only excuse for missing a lecture was illness. After lunch we had a short rest, and then went to the hospital wards, the laboratories, the library or private study. There were always studies and homework and we would exchange notes and copy pictures from one another if we missed a point in class.

I was shocked by the physiology lecture discussing how embryos develop! The physical details of women's organs and the formation of ova and sperm was a real eye-opener for most of us boys. We had no previous knowledge of this side of human life. The girls were very quiet and embarrassed in the class. Gradually we all came to terms with it.

I was supported financially by Bauji for my food and accommodation, but there was little money left for visiting the cinema or shopping or for any luxury espresso coffee or games. I was lucky to hear of a family near to Medical School who were looking for a private tutor for their daughters. I applied and got the job to teach physics, biology and maths for two hours, twice a week. They paid me well. The income was very helpful as I always found money got me to places I would otherwise not be able to go. I was able to mingle with all my friends who could easily afford all the amenities and luxuries, as they came from rich families.

Sometimes in an evening we would leave college and go to the Kwality restaurant on the outskirts of town for an espresso coffee. In the coffee lounge I saw for the first time dances other than Indian Dance. I saw cha-cha, rhumba and the tango!

One night my friends and I were outside under the stars enjoying the hot night. We were talking and playing games and we invited all in Block A to join us. A few would not join the group. I felt mischievous and in need of some fun. I put a copper coin in my lamp holder, causing an electrical short and plunged Block A into complete darkness. No-one could study until the short was mended the following day. My practical joke was intended to compel everyone to enjoy each other's company, join us and listen to our jokes. My trick really worked and most students joined in and went out for a late night film show or gossiped in the middle of block. Next day everybody found out about my mischief and some of my friends said: "Well done!"

There was a tradition in medical college every now and again to have a picnic for the whole class. With food prepared in the mess, we set off in the college bus. We rode into the countryside and eventually stopped by an orchard near to the riverbank. We would sit in a circle and each one of us would have to perform some party piece. Each act was appreciated with clapping and laughter. We took a boat on the river, singing Bollywood songs as we punted along. The picnics were all the more interesting as it was a great opportunity to get to know the girls.

The first time that I saw the Golden Temple at Amritsar I thought it looked very impressive. There it stands, gleaming with a real gold dome, in the middle of its man-made lake. The only way into the Gurdwara is by way of the bridge over the lake. We took our shoes off and covered our heads with handkerchiefs. We made our way inside to the main area where the Granth Sahib is kept. There we knelt and listened to the readings taken from it. They are read aloud from sunrise to sunset. A holy man with his blue robes and magnificent long snow-white beard constantly waved a white fan from side to side over the holy book. The whole atmosphere around the Gurdwara was of beauty, peace and harmony.

We came to the food hall and had *langer*, made from a mixture of pulses and lentils. There was salad and pickle. The food was served in stainless steel bowls. *Halwa,* made from flour, oil and raw sugar, was dessert. The drink is always cold water served in a stainless steel mug. All this is free to all pilgrims. It is made, served, and the plates washed, by Sikhs, from the highest to the lowest. Thus a cabinet minister might serve a rickshawala; a millionaire might serve a lavatory cleaner.

The dark interior caught a shaft of light every now and again, hinting and glinting at the gold decorations within the walls and alcoves. We emerged blinking into the sunlight. We had a dip in the lake and said some prayers. With the evening sunset, a dazzling light shone on the gold dome and reflected in the lake. The Gurdwara, the lake and the surrounding buildings appeared transported into another dimension not of this world.

The first trip was so wonderful we vowed to visit the Golden Temple on Sunday once every month, our day off from college.

The friends I made at medical college have remained life-long friends. We have an association through which we keep in touch and hold annual get-togethers, across three continents: India, North America and in Britain.

34: Delhi Doctor

I QUALIFIED FROM AMRITSAR in the winter of 1964. A number of my class fellows and I took house jobs in hospitals in Delhi. I joined The All India Institute of Medical Sciences, a very prestigious institution for training. A long established hospital, it was nevertheless a mass of new buildings with extensive facilities. As newly qualified doctors, we showed off, rushing along the corridors and stalking onto the wards, stethoscopes dangling round our necks. We wore ties, even on hot summer days. We were never without medical equipment kit which bulged in our white coats, whilst a row of pens, blue, black and red, sat in a regimental row, in the top pocket.

Our working hours were not fixed but we usually started at 7am and finished at about 6pm. We spent most of our time in the hospital as we were on duty on alternate days and nights, a one-in-two rota. There were interesting lectures by well-known professors and overseas visiting academics.

I was very impressed by the vast engine that was the working hospital; I was proud to be a cog in the machinery, and felt humbled by suffering humanity's trust in my very shaky skills. An excellent junior doctor's mess with a bar, facilities for sports and games and a lively social life made them very happy days.

In the summer we slept on the roof of the mess. Draped in our mosquito nets, we could still see a beautiful view of stars and moon. The Hospital was very close to the airport. Everything from jets to biplanes flew over there. We would lie up on the roof, excitement gathering as planes roared overhead on their way to and from Delhi's Palam airport. None of us had taken an air flight in our life, and it was great to be so close to these roaring magic carpets from far-flung places.

I had always had an interest in flying, and my friend TC Jain and I took up gliding at nearby Saftarjung Airport .We flew a number of flights with an instructor and then we graduated to flying solo. To look down and see Delhi from high in the air was a great experience. My younger brother Kuckoo visited me for a few days. He was interested in my new life. Kuckoo was by then six feet tall and all my friends thought he was my *elder* brother.

I moved on to Irwin Hospital in the middle of Delhi, near Connaught Place. I took up bone surgery, orthopaedics. It was with great emotion and a heart full of thanks that I walked the very same ward and "gowned up" in the very same operating theatre where I had been operated upon by Professor Robert Roaf, 13 years before. I met some of the nursing staff who had looked after me as a child. Some still remembered me.

The job was particularly busy, as I had to cover the Casualty Department, the busiest in the whole of Delhi, as it serves Delhi city and the surrounding countryside as well. I saw and treated acute emergency cases. I learned to make decisions quickly and think on my feet. My Father and Mother were very proud when they visited me in the hospital, especially as it was the same hospital where I was operated on as a child.

My cousin Asha and her husband, Major Harbans Lal Saluja, lived in the Delhi Cantonment. I often visited them on my day off and spent time with Rita, Renu and Kumkum, their daughters. "Shall we go and see a film, then maybe to the Standard restaurant in Connaught Place?" I usually said, and I knew the answer would always be: "Yes!" But I wanted to widen my horizons. I explored the possibility of leaving India and going to America. I took and passed the ECFMG exam so I could take an internship in America.

So, fully qualified and with skills in medicine, surgery and obstetrics, I was ready for the world. Most of our Professors had taken post-graduate education in England, so they and the government of the UK encouraged us to go there. Most of my friends decided to go to the UK and I followed suit. I applied for a UK visa which, as there was a shortage of doctors there, was given without further ado.

As a House Officer, I was paid only pocket money. I needed to raise the funds for my air fare to the UK. So I took a job in The Department of Health in Delhi Administration and was posted to the Tuberculosis Hospital in Mehrauli as an assistant surgeon. It was a very busy and overcrowded hospital. TB was rampant as the conditions for communicating the disease were ideal with the overcrowding and undernourishment, together with the fact that, unlike most microbes, TB thrives in sunlight. Clinics were overcrowded; and we had to conduct lung examinations, which entailed passing a metal tube down the windpipe, without the benefit of a general anaesthetic.

I spent very little of my wages and eventually I had enough to buy a ticket to the UK – one way. I was allowed to bring £3 sterling. So when I finally arrived, I had only a small suitcase containing my qualification certificates and stethoscope, a change of clothes, my new shoes and that £3 in my pocket.

35: Goodbye to My Family

SO. I HAD DECIDED I wanted to go to England. My parents were proud and happy about my going abroad for studies but anxious that I should not be away too long. They agreed that two years in England would be sufficient to gain post-graduate experience. My family knew I had decided to remain single until I had completed my education. Nevertheless, before my departure, Beeji was very anxious to find a girl as my future bride so she would be waiting for me on my return. Bauji and Beeji arranged a havan blessing for me at the temple. Relations came from near and far to wish me well in my studies and give me blessings; they joked that I would very likely marry a *memsahib* from London, settle and have a family and they might never see me again.

I left for England in June 1966. Relatives and friends arrived at Palam Airport in Delhi to bid me farewell. I was overwhelmed by the number who gathered to garland me with flowers and wish me well. I thought how close my family circle was and I was somewhat embarrassed at the fuss being made of me. "Good luck to him, he'll marry an English girl and we can visit in few years' time!" Kamlesh and Davinder joked to my brothers. Mohan Singh, our neighbour, seeing Mother's eyes well up, whispered reassuringly in her ear: "Don't you worry. He'll be back in no time with his post-graduate degree."

Following Indian custom, I bent and touched the feet of Bauji and Beeji as a mark of respect. My brothers and sister, cousins and friends, bear-hugged me until I was breathless. I waved one last goodbye and turned to board the Middle Eastern Airline flight to Bombay, as it was then called. I was exhilarated and interested in everything I saw.

Now I was set for England, I thought a lot about the family that I was about to leave. First of all, Beeji who was a tremendous mother. Her own mother died when she was only three years old, and her elder sister took her into her care. She had the ability to assess a situation as if she had a sixth sense and was very determined to improve our lot when we became refugees after the Partition. It was Mother who had asked for an appointment with our school principal and argued the case for our school fees to be waived so that we had free education. She was the driving force in our family and could be relied upon to provide an amicable solution to most problems.

She had a network of family and friends throughout the country, particularly in Meerut and Delhi, making her a very useful person to know if a good match for a girl or boy was being arranged.

She was politically active and canvassed for any candidate who agreed to deliver the services the neighbourhood needed or wanted. She was a member of the women's section of the Congress Party, and attended many rallies, persuading members of parliament to improve local community facilities. We children teased her, announcing that she would make a very good home minister. She and Shashi were very close and always closed ranks against us boys and Bauji when it came to card games.

"Let us give these boys a good game. We will play calmly and show what we are made of and let them do the shouting and I hope they don't cheat," Shashi would say to Bauji.

"This is emotional blackmail. We are trusting players and would give you a fair game," Raj would whisper to Shashi. We could win the game; but to keep it going for longer, we would help the girls with some of the moves.

Bauji was a kind and loving father who also spent a lot of time helping our friends and neighbours. He was a true gentleman, mild-mannered, honest and unfailingly kind to us all. Unfortunately these attributes did not help him in business. He was a *jamidar*, a gentleman farmer, but during the Partition he had been forced to leave our 60,000-acre farm behind in the newly-created Pakistan and flee for his life. Once settled in Meerut, he had set up a wholesale coal delivery firm. He regarded the world of business as unprincipled and corrupt, so spent a great deal of time in the Arya Samaj Hindu temple doing its accounts or administrative work. I spent many happy hours with him down at the freight yard where his wagons filled with coal came shunting and clanking into the railway sidings.

He was not worldly-wise but scrupulously honest in his business. He had amazing patience and was never cross with anyone. He went to extraordinary lengths to help others. He counted not the cost nor the time involved when he saw someone need a helping hand. Sometimes, according to Mother, we didn't get as much of his time as we needed – he could never say no to anyone. Neighbours who could not read or write would come round to our house bringing documents for interpretation or forms for filling. We were shooed out to play, as his help was always given discreetly, with patience and humility. He certainly did not want our interest and curiosity, all ears and eyes, or our noisy comings and goings, racing through the house, when an embarrassed person knocked on the door needing help. Beggars in need of a meal could be sure of a few annas from the cash that Bauji would scrape together from the little that we had for our own needs.

"I'm going to Arya Samaj to do the accounts. I'll be back in a couple of hours." But he was always late and Beeji had dinner waiting for him. When he returned, he would say: "I'm sorry; so-and-so isn't well, so I took him to see the doctor and did his bit of shopping." On other occasions Bauji would be away for hours helping a labourer at the coalyard to present a case to a solicitor or even in court to the judge.

When Pakistan was torn off from the top of India, the countries divided on religious principles. There were many people trapped on the 'wrong' side, who for one reason or another could not escape. They were caught up in the usual atrocities and bloodshed that history repeats over and over again. Bauji was involved through our local temple in the rehabilitation of Hindu women who had been raped and tortured in Pakistan before escaping over the border. "When these women return to our community," he said, "they will be treated with respect as mother, sister or daughter. Nobody shall raise anything about what happened to them during Partition." He, together with Mother, was very vocal in their support.

Then there was big brother Brij. He was seven years older than me; and, being the eldest son, his was a position of respect. He got the first bicycle in the family as soon as he was in senior school. We younger ones thought him very mature and wise, and he was a leader among his friends He was always quiet, a brother of few words, but always kind and gentle; and, even when young, was considered to be very learned.

In early childhood Brij was slim, tall with dangly legs that we used to tickle as they would stick out of the charpoy. He wore short trousers with his tee-shirt hanging over. He was conscious of his figure and looked smart with his new clothes which he always got first. He was generally quiet in the family but on occasion made up for it by losing his cool.

As a teenager he was six foot tall, with a large forehead and broad nose. He was very well groomed with long flowing hair and well-shaped moustache. Later on he became very keen on beards and kept a Bulganin beard for a long time. He put on weight with time and his hair started receding on both sides of the forehead and he had round-framed spectacles. He achieved a BA and an MA in Economics with excellent grades, and then started looking for work. We had a close relationship with our cousin Raj Kalra, and Brij joined him, far away in Assam, to work as manager in a plywood factory there. Thousands of miles away to the east, Assam has the highest rainfall in the world so naturally is covered in forests and is very green. There were thousands of tea plantations.

Eventually Brij was promoted and posted to the Hindustan Mountains Institute as a director. He had always been interested in climbing and outdoor pursuits, and now was in charge of the development and advancement of mountaineering equipment, working very closely with Tenzing Norgay, the Nepalese who had, with Edmund Hillary, reached the summit of the holy and sacred *Jommalongu* (Everest) in 1953. When Brij visited us at home, he would entertain us for hours with stories of adventure in the mountains, thrilling us with his first-hand accounts of the dangerous situations needed to enable them to test new equipment.

Tenzing Norgay was the field training director in the institute and they spent a lot of time camping in the mountains. One day Brij said: "I'll tell you a true story about Edmund Hillary. He had a narrow escape when they were out training on the south face of Jommalongu. I think he was moving loads up to the next camp one day, when the ice gave way and a huge deep crevasse opened up and he slipped in. Tenzing, who was following on behind, had dug his ice-axe into the snow; quick as a flash he put the rope round it and held on to the rope with all his might. Edmund Hillary dangled on the end of the rope looking down into the fathomless blue crevasse, whilst Tenzing hauled him to safety."

Brij was very impressed with Tenzing's religious fervour. He was a Buddhist, and as such did not injure or kill any creature. He always prayed for the team's success and safety before he set out on any climbs. Brij helped to set up the Himalayan Mountaineering Institute, a group that organises mountaineering and adventure courses for teenagers to develop a new capacity and skill in mountain climbing. We were all very proud of Brij. And when he brought home a photograph showing him high up in the mountains with Tenzing, it had pride of place on our sitting room mantelpiece.

Then there was my sister Shashi. As the only girl amongst a family of boys, Shashi was very shy, reserved and clingy to Mother. Shashi was a very attractive girl with poise and a slim figure. Heads would turn on the street but she was not conscious of it. She blossomed in time and became self-assured, confident, and joined the NCC, the Territorial Army, and went to Kashmir as a volunteer to teach young children.

Shashi was 18 months younger than me and I was always trying to do things to impress or scare her. She was very good at screaming, and that caused laughter all round. Even though I did tease her most of the time, I was always there to look after Shashi and usually escorted her to visit her girlfriends, staying around until she was ready to come home. I was shy with these girls to begin with. But, thanks to Shashi's introduction and the fact that I was her brother, I gradually gained more confidence in talking with them and started teasing them, just as I did her. She would encourage me. "Don't worry about them, they won't bite you and they really like you and would not mind going out with you."

We would play games like chase and catch, and I would tickle the back of some girl's neck if I could reach that far, to be rewarded by screams from them all. We amused ourselves like this until Shashi went to Intercollege to do her economics degree. She was also very musical and became a very good sitar player. My abiding memory of Shashi is of her being adamant that she would knit me a polo-neck sweater. She did in time, and I treasured it – in spite of the fact that it was loose and I teased her, saying that she made me look like King Kong. She took it in good heart and replied that she had *intended* to make me look fat.

The brother-sister relationship is very strong in India and our parents impressed upon us the fact that it is a brother's place to take care of his sister. Shashi was the only sister we five brothers had. She was very close to Beeji, from whom she learned cookery and how to run a home. She was not spoiled, even though she was the only girl. When we brothers grew older, it was always Shashi we brought presents for, every time we came home.

36: Doctor Mehta Who Makes It Better

I BOARDED THE PLANE at Delhi and went to Bombay, as people then called it, and stayed overnight at The Sun and Sand Hotel. I had never been inside an hotel, let alone a five-star like The Sun and Sand. The doorman, a monumentally tall and magnificent Sikh, in his uniform and turban of royal blue, gold braid on his shoulders and across his expansive chest, saluted me in. A huge chandelier twinkled above the cool and cavernous reception hall. The rich hum of classical sitar music floated on the air and I could see a girl playing it, sitting on a floor cushion, her silk sari draped around her. I was caught by a whiff of her expensive perfume as I passed on my way to reception desk.

My room was on the seventh floor, so I enjoyed the view of the sweeping curve of Bombay beach. After refreshing myself, I went down for dinner in the subdued light of The Garden Restaurant. I ordered comforting and familiar Punjabi food. I ate alone at a table in the corner. By the time I returned to my room, darkness had fallen and the view from the window was of millions of diamond lights, the famed *maharani's necklace,* twinkling and flickering around Bombay harbour. I left for the airport three hours before the flight time in order to complete the passport and visa checks and to get my vaccinations. That afternoon I boarded my flight to London.

Heathrow Airport at last! And I made my way to the lavatory! Unfortunately, the signs on the lavatory doors were unfamiliar and I went to the ladies' by mistake. I locked the small cubicle door and turned around to see a lavatory bowl raised up off the floor like a throne. I had never come across this arrangement in my life – I was used to a hole in the ground. I stood on the seat and squatted down, balancing precariously. As I stood at the sink later to wash my hands, I could feel indignant stares and a few mutterings. One woman tossed her scarf around her neck and said: "You're in the wrong toilet, sonny."

"I am so sorry, it is my mistake!" I hurried out of the ladies, covered in embarrassment.

I arrived in London in the early morning. I looked up at the sky and it was a beautiful shade of grey. A summer mist hung over the place, a very pleasant relief from the steamy cauldron I had just left. Only trouble was: I didn't realise it was likely to last for the next 40 years! My cousin Narinder met me. Narinder lived in a bedsit in Bayswater and had been in London for two years. He worked in the High Commission of India in Aldwych. I had a rest, and Narinder and I had a meal in the afternoon. We walked along Bayswater Road towards Hyde Park Corner. The roads struck me as very quiet and orderly, no car horns, no cows, just free-flowing traffic. I liked the black London cabs and the red buses.

We strolled along to the Serpentine Pub in Hyde Park. There was a lake with ducks and swans. The flower borders were ablaze with colour, and I sniffed the perfumed air. The evening was warm and humid, but not as hot as in India. It was cloudy and there was a light shower as we were going back to the bedsit.

Narinder lived in an eight-by-ten-foot room with a large casement window overlooking the street at one end and a door to the corridor at the other. The room had a high ceiling and decorated cornices. The houses in the area had been grand at one time, but now the whole street was a rabbit warren of little cubes. Toilets were shared with six other bedsitters in the corridor. Narinder had an electric cooking stove in his room, which he used to cook Indian food as he could not adjust to typical English food. We had baked beans on toast but sprinkled with chilli sauce. He kindly gave me his bed and slept on a mattress on the floor. "I will give you a fantastic typical English breakfast!" he said whilst grooming to go to his work at the Commission. He made an egg and bacon sandwich. I must say breakfast was delicious. I had never eaten bacon before.

Narinder was always smartly dressed in a dark suit, a white shirt and winkle-picker shoes. He wore sunglasses as soon as we got up, indoors or out, sunshine or no. "When you speak to English people, you should talk at a very slow pace as they will not catch your Indian accent," he advised. He punctuated his conversation with "thank ya" and "please" and "excuse *meee*," and even "oh, darn't mind if ah do." He never spoke like that in India. He spoke with a twang which I later realised was Cockney. The next day I collected all my papers and made my way to the General Medical Council, where I registered. I then visited the British Medical Association and applied for jobs as a junior house officer. I had an interview and was asked to come back in two days time.

I met up with Narinder and we went to the Standard Indian Restaurant in Bayswater. We arrived back at the bedsit and were invited by Mrs Bolling, the landlady, for drinks and snacks. The first time I had met Mrs Bolling, a cigarette was stuck to her lower lip and a long ash was hanging, ready to drop. She had worn a patterned overall and had rollers in her hair, covered by a scarf. But later I could see she was blonde and in her mid-sixties. With her kind and open face, wrinkled around her eyes and neck, she grabbed Narinder and said to me: "I am very fond of Narinder, he is like my son."

Mrs Bolling had a beautiful daughter, Marcasita. She was a big-busted bottle blonde with shiny long hair in a bird nest hairdo. She wore make-up put on with a spade and trowel. She wore bright red lipstick and well defined eyebrows. There was a twinkle in her blue eyes, surrounded by their long sweeping artificial eyelashes, which hinted that Marcasita liked to have fun. She wore high-heeled long leather boots. My eyes strayed to her low-neck dress and mini-skirted bottom. She came straight over and embraced me in a tight hug. *To welcome me to England*! She said. Her perfume was strong.

"It's gonna be good to 'ave a doctor in the 'ouse," she smiled, "ya can listen to me chest and tell me I'm in love." She laughed. "I want ya ta 'ear me 'eartbeat goin' boom boom with ya stethoscope." I was taken aback. I was not accustomed to advances from beautiful young women. Marcasita certainly knew how to break the ice and make me feel at home in a foreign country. She was charming and was just being her usual friendly self.

Marcasita wanted to know all about me and I talked about my plans. We had beer and snacks. Marcasita was in a jovial mood and, of course, she wanted to do the "Oh, doctor I'm in trouble" song, with me doing the Peter Sellers "well, goodness gracious me" bit, whilst she was Sophia Loren. She insisted I bring out my stethoscope and listen to her chest. It was an enjoyable evening. After that, Marcasita made a point of saying "Doctor I'm in trouble" every time I saw her.

The next day I went to the BMA house and was offered a job in St Mary's Hospital in Paddington. This was a very busy hospital and the queues of patients waiting for treatment in every department were very long. For the first two days I followed my mentor, the registrar, to get used the routine of my new job in my new country. On my evening off, I decided to visit Narinder in Bayswater. I turned out of the main hospital gates and walked down the road. It was a fine July evening and the sun shone with an amber glow.

Tottering along the pavement, a young girl wearing a mini-skirt and flimsy top came towards me. She had an unlit cigarette in her mouth. She then walked alongside me and asked "'Ave ya got a light?" I politely lit her cigarette. "Where d'ya live?" she enquired.

"I just started a new job in the hospital, I live in doctors' residence," I said, with a hesitant wave of my arm.

"I'm always around 'ere, ah could come to ya room any time you want!" she generously replied.

"I'm sorry, I'm going to visit my cousin in Bayswater," I said politely.

She winked and blew an airy kiss at me. When I related the incident to Narinder, he was not surprised and said: "Watch out! There are loose girls everywhere around Paddington!"

In the Doctors' Mess, excitement was at fever pitch about the football World Cup. I had never seen a television before in my life. The pitch and the faces of players came on screen, then the full live game! There was a lot of discussion about the teams among us as we congregated in front of the television set for the match. I think, in those early days, I must have spent most of my spare time watching football matches.

The match was delayed, due to rain, but was resumed within an hour – which I found interesting. In India, if it rains, it pours for days and there is no chance of restarting the game the same day. We bought England flags to wave in the Doctors' Mess. Car drivers had the England flag fluttering from their aerials. This was an exciting time. The match between Argentina and England was a bit controversial and we all knew England was the better team. In the end, as every English person knows, England reached the World Cup Final and played against West

Germany. Everyone was given the day off to cheer England. There were hours of pre-match discussions among the football pundits and excitement at Wembley Stadium. We congregated around the television set in the Doctors' Residence.

We bought two crates of beer so that we didn't run out of drink. The match was very exciting and, with England winning, there was a controversial decision by the referee which disallowed a German goal. Then Geoff Hurst scored another goal to seal England's victory. We went wild with excitement!

"I knew it!" we said. We congratulated each other with back-slapping, cheering and punching the air. Then we had yet another drink. Everybody felt so proud of England when the World Cup was presented to Bobby Moore.

"Moore's the best!" we said. The England Captain and his team took a lap of honour, carrying the Cup high around Wembley Stadium. The whole country was euphoric. I began to see just how popular football is in the west. It was as if the whole country had gone mad. I wondered if the English always behaved like this. A few days later there was a parade of the Cup when the players went around the streets of London in an open-topped bus.

I learned a great deal at St Mary's Hospital and applied for a Senior House Officer Job at Worcester Royal Infirmary. I went to the railway station and asked for a ticket to go to Wor-*ces*-ter. The ticket master said: "You mean Wooster!" So I attended the interview, secured the job, and learned how to say *Worcester*.

I started the following month, and was given temporary accommodation in the Assistant Matron's flat. It had one bedroom, a sitting room, kitchen and hall, and a bathroom. Showers are the usual way to wash in India and I had access to one in St Mary's. The Assistant Matron's flat had no shower, but it did have a bath. *I never had a bath before* so I decided to try it.

I filled the bath to the brim and got in. The water spilled over the rim of the bath and on to the carpet. It poured through the floor and through the ceiling below. It poured into *Matron's* flat. Cleaners were sent to mop up as much as they could. In spite of their efforts, a new carpet had to be put on the bathroom floor. I was very upset but the hospital manager was very kind about the whole incident.

"Don't you worry about it," Mary the cleaner winked, "I'll dry it up."

"This old carpet needed a replacement anyway," the hospital manager said.

Worcester is a beautiful old town standing on the river Trent. The Infirmary is in the centre of the town and it was possible to walk from the hospital, along the banks of the river to Worcester Cricket Club. I often went to see the County Matches on my day off. I saw Basil D'Oliveira, David Graveney and the Nawab of Pataudi. And I medically attended to some of the players in the accident and emergency department.

"Anyone want to come for a swift half with me?" I'd enquire with my head round the door of the doctors' sitting room. On our nights off, we would explore the pubs of Worcester; sometimes we went further field into the country pubs in Broadway and around the Malvern Hills. Research, we called it, to get the real feel of the pubs. There were parties in the doctors' mess and we celebrated on any excuse.

My sister Shashi had been married in 1965 to Harbans Narula and they were very happy. They were expecting their first child when I left for England. Narinder came with the joyous news that they had a little boy, Sunny, and everything was well. I went shopping in Mothercare for gifts on my next day off and sent a parcel of baby items that I knew would not be available in India. Two weeks later Narinder phoned to say that Shashi was very ill and in hospital. He phoned again later to tell me Shashi had died of a cerebral thrombosis. It was heartbreaking. She was 22 years old and Sunny was two weeks old. I was set to return to India but my Consultant was very kind and reassuring. He said that I would not be any help by going back home to India. He said I should try to achieve my goal in England. I spent some time with my cousin in London and then returned to Worcester and immersed myself in my job.

In the Orthopaedic Ward we covered both adults and children. Charmaine, a young lady of sixteen, was admitted with a compound fracture of the leg after falling from a horse. She had an operation and was kept in hospital for a few weeks.

Charmaine was a very good patient and the doctors and nurses made a fuss of her. She wrote a poem about all the staff and she gave a card to me saying: "To Doctor Mehta, who makes it better."

When she was discharged, her parents came to collect her. They asked Sister to call me. "You've been so good to our Charmaine; she thinks the world of you. We'd like you to come over for tea." Charmaine's parents sent a taxi to collect me from the hospital and I had tea with them at their farm. I was astounded when, as I made my way to go, Charmaine said: "Hang on a minute, Doctor; we've got something for you." Charmaine's father emerged from the barn with a white Pekingese puppy dog in his hands.

"I can't accept this," I stammered, "who'll look after it, take it for walks, when I'm on duty all day and night?"

They insisted I must accept it. "The maids'll look after him for you! You just need to enjoy him."

And so Tiger came to live with me. I made him a bed in a basket underneath my sink and he shared my room. The maids were very pleased to look after Tiger. He was so white, he was almost invisible in the snow except for his coal black eyes and wet black nose.

I needed to attend a residential course in preparation for my primary fellowship exam at the Royal College of Surgeons of England. I did not know how to manage with Tiger. As I was still friendly with Mrs Bolling and Marcasita in London, I took Tiger and gave him to them and went for the course.

A few weeks later, I made enquiries as to the whereabouts of Professor Robert Roaf, my hero and my inspiration. For eighteen years I had held the memory of him in my heart, and now I wanted to say "thank you" personally. He was in Liverpool. I arranged with his secretary to see him.

He was a half-remembered Great Man who had been there to save me years ago, when I was desperate and in need of help. Professor Roaf had, by his skill and experience, saved me from a one-armed life of disability and poverty. I needed to meet, just once more, the man who was the reason for my chosen path in life, the man who shaped my destiny. I needed to thank him personally. I polished my shoes, Brylcreemed my hair and folded my blue mackintosh over my arm. I set off on the early morning train from Worcester to Liverpool. A bus to the Royal Orthopaedic Hospital went through the wet streets of Liverpool that late September morning.

I was escorted by his secretary to the Professor's office. Robert Roaf stood up from behind his desk and shook hands. *He did not remember me!* When I reminded him of the only child in the adult ward at Irwin Hospital, the eight-year-old who followed him on his ward rounds, his face beamed. He said: "Yes! I remember! I *do* remember a man with hopeful eyes, carrying a small boy, infected elbow joint, badly infected, maggots crawling in and out osteomyelitis all over."

He went on: "Some people said amputation would be the best thing, and done quickly, too." Professor Roaf looked at me closely. "They thought: *if* the boy recovered, we could fit a very good false arm, a hook to pick things up..." He slapped his head. "Well, who'd have thought...? I'll be damned! I'm so glad we didn't do it! I should've known you were trailing after me for some reason!"

The function he had restored to my fingers, the arm he had drained of pus and the ambition he had inspired in me against all odds, I put to good use. I was going to be a surgeon. I was joining his profession. The two of us examined my crooked elbow with the gunstock deformity and the three huge scars. There in his office, the pale northern sunshine streamed in through the long window and shone on the leather chairs, the bookcases and the portraits of bygone orthopaedic surgeons that hung on the wall. The sun shone on the both of us and my heart was overwhelmed with gratitude. India was six thousand miles away and we were recalling half-forgotten memories from fifteen years ago.

I enquired about Sister Margaret. "She retired last year and moved near her family," he said, "I'll let her know her little Hindi teacher has arrived in London, and he's a qualified doctor!"

He took both my hands in his and congratulated me on achieving my medical degree. He wished me well and insisted I let him know of my progress in surgery.

The Professor was a warm and inspiring person. I have great memories of him which I cherish to this day. I kept in touch with him until he retired and moved away.

L - #0128 - 130522 - CO - 229/152/10 - PB - DID3312624